Medicine, Health and Social Welfare in Post-1

Historical Studies of Contemporary China

Edited by

Thomas DuBois (*Beijing Normal University*)
Huaiyin Li (*The University of Texas at Austin*)

VOLUME 5

The titles published in this series are listed at *brill.com/hscc*

Medicine, Health and Social Welfare in Post-1949 China

Edited by

Liping Bu
Xiaoping Fang

Translated by

Zhang Xiaoqin and Li Yiyang

Proofread by

Luo Hongyan

BRILL

LEIDEN | BOSTON

经典中国国际出版工程
China Classics International

This book is a result of the co-publication agreement between Social Sciences Academic Press and Koninklijke Brill BV. These articles were selected and translated into English from the Chinese journal, *History Studies of Contemporary China* (《当代中国史研究》 Dangdai Zhongguo shi yanjiu), edited by 李正华 Li Zhenghua and sponsored by the Institute of Contemporary China, Chinese Academy of Social Sciences. The translation has received financial support from the Innovation Program of the Chinese Academy of Social Sciences.

The Library of Congress Cataloging-in-Publication Data is available online at https://catalog.loc.gov
LC record available at https://lccn.loc.gov/2025018154

Typeface for the Latin, Greek, and Cyrillic scripts: "Brill". See and download: brill.com/brill-typeface.

ISSN 2352-7919
ISBN 978-90-04-73798-3 (hardback)
ISBN 978-90-04-73799-0 (e-book)
DOI 10.1163/9789004737990

This book is printed on acid-free paper and produced in a sustainable manner.

Contents

Tables

Editors' Note on Translation

Chapters of this volume were originally published in the journal, *Historical Studies of Contemporary China*. They were translated from Chinese into English by Zhang Xiaoqin and Li Yiyang and proofread by Luo Hongyan. Certain Chinese terms of social and health programs have variations of translation across the chapters, though editors of this volume have attempted to bring consistency within a chapter via copyediting. As Chinese medicine is an ongoing medical field with continuing development, we decide to use Chinese medicine instead of traditional Chinese medicine for the translation of *zhongyi* but retain TCM in such terms as TCM practitioners for the convenience of use.

CHAPTER 1

The Establishment and Development of a Socialist Healthcare and Epidemic Prevention System in the People's Republic of China

Hu Kefu[*]

Abstract

The socialist healthcare system in China, which had been built amidst the great transformation of the society, expanded rapidly as a result of the Chinese government's vigorous promotion. The glaring inadequacy of healthcare in rural areas was effectively addressed, with spectacular results achieved in healthcare for women and children nationwide, and improved access to healthcare in ethnic minority regions that contributed to their social progress. In the meantime, a nationwide epidemic prevention system was established, producing a far-reaching effect on the all-round development of the country's healthcare.

Keywords

socialist healthcare – epidemic prevention system – healthcare establishment and development

As an important measure of a country's or a region's overall strength, the provision of modern healthcare services points to the social progress, living environment, and quality of life in the country or the region. It also has a significant impact on its international competitiveness and image. The establishment and continuous growth of China's socialist healthcare reflect the changes in the broader social context over the years and epitomize the pioneering work the country has done in promoting progress in the material, political, cultural and ethical aspects. Research of healthcare in light of contemporary Chinese

---

* Hu Kefu, born in 1954, is a member of the Editorial Department of *Contemporary Hebei*, a journal run by the Hebei Academy of Social Sciences.

 | DOI:10.1163/9789004737990_002

history is of great value, for healthcare is an important part of the ambitious goal defined at the 16th National Congress of the Communist Party of China (CPC) – building China into a moderately prosperous society in all respects by 2020. Moreover, such research will help address the country's practical need for a modern healthcare sector against the backdrop of an information age. It will facilitate the work towards universal access to healthcare resources and equitable sharing of the benefits brought by the advances in medical sciences.

1 Promoting Healthcare with Emphasis on Rural Areas, Ethnic Minorities and Vulnerable Groups

The five years since the founding of the People's Republic of China (PRC) in 1949 was the formative period for China's healthcare sector. The health policy, formulated under the leadership of the CPC Central Committee and on the basis of the country's reality and the tasks for the period, required health workers to "serve the vast majority of the people, focus on preventive measures, unite Western medicine and Chinese medicine, and launch a mass movement of health". This policy had profound implications for healthcare and embodied the country's practices and fundamental principles in building the institutional framework of socialism.

For the newly founded People's Republic of China, industrialization was both its immediate goal and the means for the nation to rise and to thrive. Healthcare, however, remained a serious challenge as it inherited very limited healthcare resources from the old regime when all the social services had to be rebuilt after the war. Just before the PRC was founded in 1949, there had been only 3,670 healthcare institutions nationwide, including 2,600 hospitals, 769 outpatient clinics and 80,000 hospital beds. Moreover, infectious, endemic and parasitic diseases had posed a serious threat to human health. In particular, the number of people suffering from schistosomiasis, malaria and filariasis alone reached seventy million, death rate stood at twenty-five per thousand percent, and the average life expectancy was only thirty-five years. In such a context, building a new socialist healthcare would be of great significance for protecting people's health, keeping up popular morale, rapidly revitalizing the economy, and consolidating the new people's democratic government.

After the founding of the PRC, under the leadership of the CPC Central Committee and Mao Zedong, the people's governments set up health departments at the central, provincial, municipal, county and town levels in a manner that was never seen before in China's history. These departments, which were entrusted with the arduous task of eliminating pests and acute diseases and protecting people's health, allowed administrative power to be effectively exercised on a national scale. The first National Health Conference held in Beijing in August 1950 put forward the goal of universal access to medical care throughout the country. At the celebration of the first anniversary of the PRC's founding held by the National Committee of the Chinese People's Political Consultative Conference (CPPCC) on September 30 that year, Premier Zhou Enlai made it clear once again that "the People's Government has decided to set up health departments in every county and district in the next few years to resolve the long-standing problem of the low level of public health."[1] It showed the resolve and determination of the CPC and the Chinese government to develop the healthcare sector in the early years of the PRC.

1.1 *Addressing the Glaring Inadequacy of Healthcare in Rural Areas*

Healthcare was grossly inadequate in rural areas before the founding of the PRC. The country had, on average, less than one hospital and less than 10 hospital beds per county among the 2,100 some counties. The First National Health Conference held in August 1950 adopted the *Decision to Fully Build and Develop Basic Level Health Organizations in the Entire Country*, which required a healthcare institution to be built in every city district and every rural town. It also required that every county must have a county hospital, every district a health station, every administrative village a health committee, and every natural village a health worker. In following up the decision, the Ministry of Health established and improved hospitals at the county (banner and autonomous county in ethnic minority areas) level, and authorized them to manage public health affairs within their counties. After that, the Ministry of Health issued the *Measures for the Organization of United Medical Institutions*, the *Provisional Rules for the Organization of County Hospital*, and the *Provisional Rules for the Organization of County District Health Stations*. In doing so, it sought to create a county-wide healthcare network that comprised the three tiers of counties, towns and villages. By the end of 1952, there had been 2,123 county hospitals (health centers) with 37,467 beds in the country. During the first Five-Year Plan period (1953–1957), district health stations evolved into district health centers in the transformation of cooperative agriculture. Modern medical science was used to directly serve the peasants for the first time in Chinese history, which counted as a giant stride in the country's endeavor to advance the material, political, cultural and ethical progress. Despite the achievements, there was still a long way to go before the inadequacy of healthcare in rural China was

1 Party Literature Research Office of the CPC Central Committee, ed. 1984. *Selected Works of Zhou Enlai* (Volume 2). Beijing: People's Publishing House. 48.

completely overcome. Mao Zedong was personally in charge of the draft of the first *National Outline for Agricultural Development from 1956 to 1965*, which included prevention, control and elimination of diseases, elimination of the four pests, hygiene and family planning. In 1965, when the urban-rural gap widened, Mao expressed his deep concerns and issued a call for "putting the focus of healthcare services in the countryside". Since then, cooperative medical care with Chinese characteristics has been rolled out in rural areas.

1.2 *Giving Priority to Healthcare for Women and Children*

Before the founding of the PRC, Chinese women had been victimized by patriarchal feudalism. There was no women's and children's healthcare in the country's poor medical care system. Statistics show that maternal mortality rate was fifteen per thousand live births and infant mortality rate was two hundred per thousand live births. A staggering infant death rate of four hundred per thousand live births was reported in Dangshan County, Anhui Province.[2] After the founding of the PRC, women gained the same social and legal status as men with a wide range of rights that were protected by the law. The CPC and the governments at all levels considered it very important to promote healthcare for women and children and identified it as a central task in the development of socialist healthcare. Women's and children's healthcare had an important impact on further liberating women in the socialist reconstruction.

In September 1949, the First Plenary Session of the Chinese People's Political Consultative Conference (CPPCC) adopted the Common Program of the CPPCC, Article 48 of which states that "Sports shall be promoted among the people. Public health and medical care shall be expanded, and attention shall be paid to the protection of health of mothers, infants and children."[3] Thereafter, the Central People's Government enacted the *Marriage Law of the People's Republic of China*. The Government Administration Council, predecessor of today's State Council, issued the *Decree on Banning the Practice of Foot-binding* and the *Regulations of the People's Republic of China on Labor Insurance*. The Ministry of Health adopted the *Directive on Strengthening Children's Healthcare*. All of those specified the measures to protect the rights and interests of women and children. The country's first national symposium on maternal and child health in August 1950 was of epoch-making significance when it decided that maternal and child health (MCH) should be promoted nationwide in a

2 Chen Haifeng, ed. 1985. *Healthcare in China*. Beijing: People's Medical Publishing House. 122.

3 Party Literature Research Office of the CPC Central Committee, ed. 1992. *Selected Important Documents Since the Founding of the People's Republic of China* (Volume 1). Beijing: Central Party Literature Publishing House. 11.

planned and step-by-step manner. During the time period, health departments across the country made all-out efforts to develop MCH services, focusing on the clinical experience of healthcare. A host of specialized MCH institutions were established successively, creating a three-tiered MCH service network of hospitals, institutes and stations. Children's healthcare was promoted by controlling the spread of acute infectious diseases among children in the first place. Active response efforts were made to contain the spread of epidemics. In October 1950, the Government Administration Council issued the *Directive on Launching the Autumn Smallpox Vaccination Campaign* and the Ministry of Health issued the *Interim Measures for Vaccination*. Smallpox vaccines were given to more than one hundred million infants and children. By the early 1960s, smallpox was eradicated in China. Moreover, huge efforts were made to develop kindergartens and nurseries and to establish polyclinics for children. As a result, a comprehensive system of healthcare for children gradually emerged, incorporating regular physical examinations, vaccination, prevention and treatment of common and frequently occurring diseases, and management of nutritional deficiencies. Those achievements led to rapid and sharp declines in maternal and infant mortality rates, which were important indicators of the level of social development in a country or region. In Beijing, for example, maternal mortality rate fell from seven per thousand live births before 1949 to 0.7 per thousand live births in 1954, while infant mortality rate dropped nearly fifty percent to 65.7 per thousand live births.[4] History shows that only socialism can completely liberate Chinese women and unleash their productive power. The development of healthcare for women and children in the early years of the PRC is an epoch-making initiative of the CPC to faithfully follow the fundamental principle of government for the people. The endeavor for women's and children's healthcare marked an enormous stride of social progress in the history of Chinese women.

1.3 *Improving Healthcare Services to Advance Social Progress in Ethnic Minority Areas*

Before the founding of the PRC, ethnic minority areas of the country lagged far behind in social and economic development, particularly in the provision of healthcare. Infectious and endemic diseases were prevalent all year round, resulting in sharp decreases in local population, with the average life expectancy of twenty to thirty years. For example, in Tibet, which accounts for about one-eighth of the country's total territorial size, there were only four clinics

4 Chen Haifeng, ed. 1985. *Healthcare in China*. Beijing: People's Medical Publishing House. 130.

and hospitals that served exclusively the three major estate-holders (government officials, nobles, and upper-ranking lamas in monasteries); while in Xishuangbanna of Yunnan Province, whose population once reached nearly two million at its peak in history, only two hundred thousand people remained before the founding of PRC, due to acute malaria epidemics.

Ethnic issues are big issues confronting all societies today. When the PRC was founded, a major test posed to the CPC and the Chinese government was to address ethnic issues properly and manage ethnic affairs successfully. The results turned out to be impressive under the leadership of CPC and Mao Zedong. Ethnic oppression, a historical legacy, was ended; equality among all ethnic groups was upheld; and regional ethnic autonomy was introduced. Moreover, on behalf of the CPC and the Chinese government, Premier Zhou Enlai promised solemnly to all minority ethnic groups that "the Central Government would strive to develop healthcare, education and economy in ethnic minority areas."[5] Hence, the introduction of healthcare services to ethnic minority areas occupied an especially important position in the PRC's endeavor to effectively manage ethnic affairs during the early years. Healthcare provision was an important venue to communicate and implement the CPC's ethnic policy, consolidate ethnic unity, and handle well ethnic relations at the time.[6]

Firstly, the Central Government offered more guidance on the development of healthcare services in ethnic minority areas to help address the deficiencies of healthcare.

The First National Conference on Healthcare for Ethnic Minorities was held in Beijing in August 1951. For the first time in Chinese history, healthcare for ethnic minorities was put on the agenda of the Central Government. The conference decided on matters of three aspects. First, healthcare institutions would be established one after another and healthcare officials would be appointed for ethnic minority areas. Second, service fees would be reduced, waived or charged according to the actual situations of regions and the specific diseases. Third, local government leaders in ethnic minority areas would strengthen the leadership in the efforts to prevent the spread of diseases and population decline. To promote the development of healthcare services in ethnic minority areas, the Culture and Education Committee of the Government Administration Council approved in December 1950 and promulgated in the

5 Party Literature Research Office of the CPC Central Committee, ed. 1984. *Selected Works of Zhou Enlai* (Volume 2). Beijing: People's Publishing House. 40.

6 Huang Guangxue, ed. 1993. *Ethnic Affairs in Contemporary China* (Volume 1). Beijing: Contemporary China Publishing House. 75.

nation the *National Health Promotion Plan for Ethnic Minorities*, the *Plan for Malaria Prevention and Treatment in Ethnic Minority Areas*, the *Plan for Prevention and Treatment of Sexually Transmitted Diseases in Ethnic Minority Areas*, and the *Plan for Promotion of Maternal and Child Health in Ethnic Minority Areas*. By the end of 1952, county-level health organizations had been established in all ethnic minority areas and the number of medical institutions had reached 1,176.[7] Before October 1, 1949, more than forty counties of Xinjiang had no medical institutions, nor in most of the rural and pastoral areas of Inner Mongolia and Qinghai. In response, the Ministry of Health restored and newly built ninety-four health institutions and twenty-four hospitals in ethnic minority areas of Xinjiang, Inner Mongolia and Qinghai between 1950 and 1951, which significantly improved the healthcare in those regions.[8]

Secondly, healthcare task forces and medical teams were sent to ethnic minority areas to provide local people with free medical services and prevent them from contracting diseases.

In the early years of the PRC, the Ministry of Health successively sent four healthcare task forces and eight epidemic prevention brigades and medical teams to Tibet, Xinjiang, Inner Mongolia, Ningxia, Gansu, Yunnan, Sichuan and other ethnic minority areas, to address the widespread epidemics in those areas. Government at the provincial level also sent various healthcare task forces, mobile medical teams, and anti-epidemic teams to ethnic minority areas to provide local people with free medical services. In particular, "forty medical teams were dispatched to northwestern and southwestern areas as well as Suiyuan and Inner Mongolia."[9] The teams concentrated their efforts, first of all, on eliminating the epidemic and endemic diseases that seriously harmed the health of ethnic minorities. They also set up stations and clinics for the prevention and control of infectious diseases. While the CPC and the Chinese government made every effort to help ethnic minorities grow their economy and improve local people's lives, they also managed to control the prevalence of various diseases there. As a result, the provision of healthcare in ethnic minority areas witnessed historic changes. Local population grew significantly in both quality and quantity. Population reproduction changed from the pattern of low growth due to high birth rates and high death rates

---

7 Huang Shuze and Lin Shixiao, ed. 1986. *Healthcare Sector in Contemporary China* (Volume 2). Beijing: China Social Sciences Press. 54.

8 Huang Guangxue, ed. 1993. *Ethnic Affairs in Contemporary China* (Volume 1). Beijing: Contemporary China Publishing House. 76.

9 Huang Guangxue, ed. 1993. *Ethnic Affairs in Contemporary China* (Volume 1). Beijing: Contemporary China Publishing House. 76.

before the founding of PRC to the pattern of high growth due to high birth rates and low death rates. At the Third Plenary Session of the Seventh CPC Central Committee in 1950, Mao Zedong talked about the work for ethnic minorities and mentioned that "there are about 30 million people of ethnic minorities in the country."[10] The population of ethnic minorities in China was over 35.32 million in 1953 when the first national census was conducted and it increased to 67.24 million in 1982 when the third national census was carried out. The average annual growth rate was 22.45 permille over twenty-nine years, much higher than the growth rate of the Han ethnic group's population during the same period – 3.65 permille. Population growth reflected social progress and prosperity in the ethnic minority areas and laid the foundation for all-round development.

The efforts to improve healthcare services in ethnic minority areas in the early years of the PRC played an irreplaceable role in promoting social progress in these areas. It stands as an ample testimony to the undeniable truth that the CPC always represents the fundamental interests of all ethnic groups and plays the core role in leading the socialist family of the Chinese nation towards common prosperity.

2 Establishing an Epidemic Prevention System for All

After the founding of the PRC, the CPC Central Committee and Mao Zedong always attached great importance to epidemic prevention. Mao issued instructions on many occasions that active efforts should be made to prevent and eliminate endemic diseases. In the winter of 1955, Mao issued a call for "the elimination of schistosomiasis", which had been rampant in China for more than two thousand years. To that end, the CPC Central Committee set up a leading group for schistosomiasis prevention and control. On June 30, 1958, *The People's Daily* carried a story about the eradication of schistosomiasis in Yujiang County, Jiangxi Province. After reading the story, Mao Zedong was so excited that he could not fall asleep that night. He picked up a pen and wrote the seven-character poem entitled *Send Away the God of Plague*.[11] Premier Zhou Enlai devoted great efforts to epidemic prevention. After the founding of the PRC, the Chinese Anti-tuberculosis Association was immediately placed under

10 Party Literature Research Office of the CPC Central Committee, ed. 1977. *Selected Works of Mao Zedong* (Volume 5). Beijing: People's Publishing House. 23.

11 Party Literature Research Office of the CPC Central Committee, ed. 1994. *Selected Poems by Mao Zedong*. Beijing: People's Literature Publishing House. 91.

the direct leadership of the Ministry of Health, making it one of the first academic medical organizations funded by the government at that time. In 1951, Zhou Enlai instructed the Ministry of Health that special attention should be paid to the fight against tuberculosis.[12] In 1952, the United States used biological weapons against China in the war against the Democratic People's Republic of Korea (DPRK, North Korea). In response, the Chinese government established the Central Epidemic Prevention Committee according to the instructions of Mao Zedong. Chaired by Zhou Enlai, the committee offered guidance on epidemic prevention efforts nationwide and achieved great success.

2.1 *Creating a Sound Organizational Structure and a Standardized Management System for Epidemic Prevention*

Plague struck northern Chahar Province (a part of Inner Mongolia today) when the PRC was just founded. On October 22, 1949, the Government Administration Council held a meeting on epidemic prevention and decided to take emergency measures to end the epidemic. A Central Anti-Epidemic Task Force was set up, along with nine anti-epidemic teams. Their responsibility was to assist local epidemic prevention efforts and go to the affected areas to end the outbreak. After that, the Ministry of Health issued the *Directive on Healthcare Development in 1950*, which explicitly required that county hospitals should make it the top priority to coordinate county-wide epidemic prevention efforts. Impressive progress on epidemic prevention was made by the end of 1950. There were eighty-eight professional anti-epidemic teams and twelve plague prevention teams, as well as local anti-epidemic teams with the participation of medical practitioners of both Chinese and Western medicine. Moreover, special prevention stations and clinics were set up in epidemic-prone areas where investigations and preventive measures were focused on schistosomiasis, malaria, kala-azar and filariasis.

To support the country's plan to develop its economy on a large scale during the first Five-Year Plan period, the Ministry of Health decided at the second National Health Conference in Beijing in December 1952 that public health should be improved to ensure the success of economic development initiatives. To that end, "the first step is to establish health organizations for manufacturing, mining and transportation sectors, focus on conducting health inspections, and experiment with the workshop responsibility system, and set up institutions to research on occupational health and diseases. The second step is to focus on the establishment of epidemic prevention stations and

12 Huang Shuze and Lin Shixiao, ed. 1986. *Healthcare Sector in Contemporary China* (Volume 1). Beijing: China Social Sciences Press. 385.

clinics and research institutes to provide special guidance and research and establish prevention and control institutions for schistosomiasis, hookworm, malaria and kala-azar."[13] In January 1953, the Government Administration Council approved the establishment of epidemic prevention stations nationwide at its 167th meeting. Since then, under the leadership of health departments at all levels, a comprehensive, professional epidemic prevention system covering both urban and rural areas was gradually formed in all administrative divisions, with epidemic prevention stations playing a major role. In Hebei Province, for example, "there were one hundred and forty epidemic prevention stations at all levels staffed by 1,939 people in 1956."[14] In addition, research organizations at all levels collaborated on epidemiological investigations and epidemic prevention studies and carried out the research and production of medicines and vaccines, which comprehensively boosted the healthcare development in the early years of the PRC.

The principle of prevention first was firmly carried out. Planned immunization was implemented since the early 1950s. People were vaccinated against cholera, typhoid fever, epidemic meningitis and other diseases. In October 1950, the Ministry of Health issued the *Interim Measures for Vaccination*, specifying that all residents in the territory of the PRC were entitled to free vaccination. In the first half of 1952, 512 million people had been vaccinated, "accounting for over eighty percent of the country's total population at the time."[15] China eradicated smallpox in the early 1960s, creating a miracle in the Chinese and world history of medicine.

At the same time, epidemic prevention began to be managed according to established rules and standards. The Ministry of Health successively issued the *Guidelines on the Prevention and Control of Schistosomiasis*, the *Guidelines on the Prevention of Cholera*, and the *Guidelines on the Prevention of Epidemic Meningitis*, among others, to make preventive measures a common and standard practice. During the first Five-Year Plan period, the Ministry of Health, alone or in conjunction with relevant authorities, issued the *Measures for Managing Soft Drinks* (the PRC's first food hygiene standard), the *Interim Measures for Managing Epidemic Prevention Stations*, the *Interim Measures for Managing Canteen Hygiene*, the *Measures for Managing Infectious Diseases*, the *Drinking*

---

13 Chen Haifeng, ed. 1985. *Healthcare in China*. Beijing: People's Medical Publishing House. 87.

14 Wang Chunran, ed. 1995. *Annals of Hebei Province: Healthcare*. Beijing: Zhonghua Book Company. 148.

15 Chen Haifeng, ed. 1985. *Healthcare in China*. Beijing: People's Medical Publishing House. 101.

Water Quality Standards, the *Provisional Hygienic Standards for the Design of Industrial Enterprises*, the *Joint Directive on Health Inspections in Urban Planning and Construction*, and the *Malaria Prevention and Control Plan*. In 1956, the State Council (formerly the Government Administration Council) issued the *Safety and Health Regulations for Factories* and the *Decision on Prevention and Control of Silica Dust Hazards in Factories and Mines*. All these suggest that the socialist epidemic prevention endeavor which mainly used preventive medicine to serve urban and rural people in the early years of the PRC had moved from early-stage exploration to a new phase of standardized system of management. Moreover, the practice of "early prevention, early detection, early diagnosis and early treatment" was promoted across the country and the creation of a modern health system was incorporated into the social and economic development plan, which led to enormous public health improvements. People's average life expectancy increased by a staggering twenty-two years over a period of eight years, from thirty-five in 1949 to fifty-seven in 1957. Such a growth rate of life expectancy set a historical record in China. It speaks volumes about the CPC's commitment to exercising power in the interests of the people and marks a milestone in the Chinese history of health promotion.

2.2 *Establishing Law-Based Quarantine Inspections at Ports of Entry*

The CPC and the Chinese government devoted much attention to quarantine inspection at ports of entry. In March 1949, the government established a maritime quarantine inspection office in Yantai. Other quarantine inspection offices were later set up in Anle (present-day Dandong), Ji'an, Tumen, Yingkou, Shanhaiguan and Huludao. After the change of administrative structure from major regions to provinces in 1953, all quarantine inspection offices were handed over to the health authorities of province, municipality and autonomous regions, except those of Beijing, Tianjin and Qinhuangdao that remained under the Ministry of Health. As the Chinese economy grew rapidly, more quarantine inspection offices were established at airports and border crossings.

In the meantime, China began quarantine inspections according to international laws and regulations, which had a far-reaching influence on the country's legal system. Relevant regulations were introduced to ensure that quarantine inspection offices would exercise their power properly to protect national health sovereignty, national interests and reputation. After the First National Quarantine Inspection Conference was held in Beijing in February 1950, the Ministry of Health issued the *Interim Measures for Transportation Quarantine*, the *Interim Measures for Civil Aviation Quarantine* and the *Interim Rules for Transportation Quarantine Flags and Garments*. The Government

Administration Council introduced the *General Rules on Baggage Inspection for Passengers and Crew Members of Import and Export Ships*, the *General Rules on Baggage Inspection for Passengers and Crew Members of Import and Export Trains*, and the *General Rules on Baggage Inspection for Passengers and Crew Members of Import and Export Airplanes*. They clearly defined what quarantine inspections at ports of entry meant and how it should be conducted.[16] In 1957, the first health law of the PRC, *Regulations on Ports of Entry Quarantine Inspection*, was adopted at the 88th meeting of the first National People's Congress' Standing Committee. The law ensured the legal basis of quarantine inspections. In March 1958, the Ministry of Health issued the *Rules for Implementing the Regulations on Ports of Entry Quarantine Inspections*, making detailed provisions on quarantine inspections at China's seaports, airports, and border crossings. As a major innovation in modern China's efforts to strengthen the legal system, the introduction of the regulations and the implementing rules had profound influence on health progress. They were the solid foundation for rapid development of quarantine inspections at ports of entry during China's era of reform and opening up.

3 Conclusion

The modernization of a country or a region depends on the all-round development of social programs. This article, therefore, tries to include the crucial issues of modernity in the research of contemporary Chinese history. First, in the 21st century, China has to develop its healthcare sector in a modern context. It needs to address the challenges posed by rapid advances in modern medical science and health technology amid economic globalization, as well as those brought by the transition from a production-focused society to a learning and consumption-focused one, from traditional to modern lifestyles, and from the need for adequate food and clothing to that for modern healthcare. Second, the strategic goal of building a moderately prosperous society in all respects set at the 16th CPC National Congress means higher requirements for the development of healthcare. In the next decade or so, China needs to diversify its investment in this sector, improve the allocation of health resources, maximize the use of such resources, and adopt a healthcare policy that covers vulnerable groups in urban and rural areas as well as in old revolutionary base areas, ethnic minority areas, border areas, and poor areas. Third, in face

16 He Jiesheng, ed. 1992. *Quarantine Inspection at Ports of Entry in China*. Beijing: People's Medical Publishing House. 18.

of high technologies and high risks of modern society, China needs to establish a healthcare service system that enables prompt response to various emergencies. Fourth, China needs to create a modern health safety net that offers everyone the access to timely, sound and people-centered healthcare and the promise of high-quality life. All of these are new issues that China needs to deal with in a new stage of development in the new century.

CHAPTER 2

Evolution of the Five-Guarantee Program in Rural China

*Song Shiyun**

Abstract

The Five-Guarantee Program, which covers those most in need in rural areas, is an important part of China's rural social security system. Amidst the industrialization, marketization and modernization processes in the past 50 years, the Program underwent three major transformations. From 1956 to 1978, it was mainly financed by collectively pooled public welfare funds and operated by production teams or brigades. From 1979 to 2001, villages and towns became the primary source of funding and material support. Since 2002, it has transitioned to a modern social security program with government as the primary source of funding while collective funds, land funds and social assistance funds as the secondary sources of funding. The changes that unfolded in the three phases were indicative of a trend towards institutionalization, standardization and law-based operation of the Program. With an increasing level of benefits and a shift from villagers' mutual assistance to public finance, the Program epitomizes China's efforts to establish a modern rural social security system.

Keywords

rural areas – beneficiaries – Five-Guarantee Program – rural social security

The Five-Guarantee Program, which covers those most in need in rural areas, is an important part of China's rural social security system. Against the backdrop of national strategies of industrialization, marketization, and modernization, the Program has gone through a transformative process over the past 50 years and played a significant role in ensuring social protection for the target groups during rural economic development and maintaining social stability, even

* Song Shiyun, Ph.D., professor in the School of Business, Liaocheng University.

 | DOI:10.1163/9789004737990_003

though it underwent difficult experiences during the political and economic reforms, especially those related to rural areas, and the limitations imposed by local socioeconomic conditions. An in-depth review of the changes in the Program and an examination of the good practices and lessons learned over the years are of great significance for China's current efforts to build a modern rural social security system suitable for China to ensure the sustainable development of economy and promote a harmonious society in rural countryside.

1 A Difficult Road in the Days When Heavy Industries Were Prioritized (1956–1978)

Since the founding of the People's Republic of China, the Communist Party of China (CPC) and the Chinese government have attached great importance to the provision of assistance to the most vulnerable groups of the population in both urban and rural areas. The Five-Guarantee Program was introduced in rural areas to cover those who had no work capability, no source of living, and no legal support, maintenance and upbringing obligations to rely on. The Program signified the high attention paid to those most in need. In the early days of the People's Republic, due to limited national resources and low levels of per capita income, and the pressing need for a solid foundation of socialist industrialization, the government did not have the ability to provide material and financial resources to support the livelihood of the most vulnerable and needed rural populations. In October and November 1953, Mao Zedong proposed the scheme of agricultural cooperatives to collectivize farming in the hope of supporting the production and livelihood of the poor farmers. He said, "About 10 percent of rural population lacked grains, and half of them are of great difficulty who are either widows, orphans or people without work ability; but the mutual-aid teams and the cooperatives can give them some help. ... The socialist transformation of private enterprises and the promotion of mutual aid and cooperatives is not merely the direction to take but the immediate task now."[1] He also said, "Some peasants are selling their land, which is not good. Although the law does not prohibit it, we should make efforts to work with them to prevent them doing so. Setting up cooperatives is the solution. Mutual-aid teams are not enough to stop peasants selling their land; only co-operatives, and big ones at that, can do so. Moreover, big co-operatives can eliminate the need of some peasants to rent out their land. A big cooperative

1 Party Literature Research Office of the CPC Central Committee, ed. 1999. *Selected Works of Mao Zedong* (Volume 6). People's Publishing House. 303–304.

of one or two hundred households can help the widows, orphans and others not provided for. Then the problem will be solved."[2] In the remarks to the book *Socialist Upsurge in China's Countryside* in 1955, Mao further pointed out: "it is the responsibility of all cooperatives to help the widows, orphans and people who have no providers or work ability (the cooperatives should admit those people as members) and help those who can work but suffer great hardship, as ways to help solve their difficulties."[3] According to Article 31 of the *National Program for Agricultural Development* (1956–1967) (Draft), which was proposed by the Political Bureau of the CPC Central Committee and released after discussion by the Supreme State Conference in January 1956, "Agricultural cooperatives should provide necessary support for the widows, orphans and members without providers, and those who have little or no work ability and the disabled veterans, to ensure that they have adequate access to food, clothes, fuel, education (for children and teenagers), and funeral services. In short, they can depend on the cooperatives in life and death."[4] On June 30, 1956, the third session of the First National People's Congress passed *The Demonstration Guidelines for Advanced Agricultural Cooperatives*, which stipulated that "agricultural cooperatives should provide appropriate support in daily living and production for the elderly, widows, orphans and members without providers, who are partially or completely unable to work. They should ensure that these members have adequate access to food, clothes, charcoals. The young children will be able to receive proper education, and the elderly will not worry about their burials once they pass away."[5] Those were the two earliest legal documents concerning the beneficiaries of the Five-Guarantee Program. Both documents defined support in terms of food, clothes, fuels, education, and funeral services (known as "Wu Bao" or "Five Guarantees"). The households or individuals eligible for these benefits are called five-guarantee beneficiaries, and the corresponding policy is known as the five-guarantee policy.[6] The Five-Guarantee

2 Party Literature Research Office of the CPC Central Committee, ed. 1999. *Selected Works of Mao Zedong* (Volume 6). People's Publishing House. 299.

3 Party Literature Research Office of the CPC Central Committee, ed. 1991. *Manuscripts by Mao Zedong after the Founding of the People's Republic* (Volume 5). Central Party Literature Press. 531.

4 Party Literature Research Office of the CPC Central Committee, ed. 1994. *Collection of Major Government Documents of the People's Republic of China* (Volume 8). Central Party Literature Press. 47.

5 Party Literature Research Office of the CPC Central Committee, ed. 1994. *Collection of Major Government Documents of the People's Republic of China* (Volume 8). Central Party Literature Press. 422–423.

6 Li Bengong and Jiang Li, eds. 1996. *Disaster Relief*. China Social Press. 196–197.

Program is the first rural social security program of the People's Republic of China, a long-term program in rural China implemented by the CPC and the Chinese government.

With the collectivization of agriculture, the cooperatives (and production brigades and production teams of the people's communes after 1958) were responsible for financing and operating the Five-Guarantee Program. They mainly provided the following assistance to the target groups. First, those who had some work capability would be offered less physically demanding jobs, such as raising pigs and goats and guarding the entrance to public spaces; and they would also be given preferences in the calculation of remuneration, known as "work points," to ensure their living standard up to that of average members. Second, those who were not able to work would be entitled to a subsidy calculated on the basis of a commune member's average working days which allowed them to claim remunerations from the cooperatives at the year-end like other commune members. Third, agricultural cooperatives would allocate money and material items directly from their public welfare funds for the food, clothes, fuel, education and funeral services to the beneficiaries per the standards stipulated by the five-guarantee policy. Fourth, the cooperatives would have designated persons to care for those who could not take care of themselves due to old age, sickness, and disabilities. For the cooperatives that could not afford to support the five-guarantee benefits because of poverty or natural disasters, the government would provide necessary financial support for the beneficiaries.

In 1957, there were 60,000 households and more than 70,000 people benefiting from the Five-Guarantee Program (each individual receiving about 50 yuan per year) in the rural areas of Shandong Province.[7] The Program covered 30,000 people in Heilongjiang Province, 19,000 of whom could do some light work.[8] More than 50,000 people in Fujian Province received five-guarantee benefits, including subsistence allowance earmarked by the Civil Affairs Department of Fujian Province.[9] In Anhui Province, the beneficiaries were divided into three types: fully supported, partially supported, and subsidized. They were given assistance in one of the following three forms: cash, in-kind assistance, and most commonly, the work-day subsidies allocated from the

---

7 Local History Compilation Committee of Shandong Province, ed. 1992. *Chronicle of Shandong Province: Civil Administration*. Shandong People's Publishing House. 212.

8 Local History Compilation Committee of Heilongjiang Province, ed. 1993. *Chronicle of Heilongjiang Province: Civil Administration*. Heilongjiang People's Publishing House. 290.

9 Local History Compilation Committee of Fujian Province, ed. 1997. *Chronicle of Fujian Province: Civil Administration*. Fangzhi Publishing House. 100.

agricultural cooperatives' public welfare fund rather than the distribution of collective income. In 1957, there were 234,524 households and 373,182 people receiving five-guarantee benefits in Anhui Province, accounting for 3.1 percent of the province's total households and 1.3 percent of the province's total population. The subsidy in Huainan and Jiangnan areas were 50 yuan per person per year for fully supported beneficiaries, 30 yuan for partially supported beneficiaries, and about 20 yuan for subsidized households (not including allowances provided by the state), while the figures were slightly lower in Huaibei area.[10] Most of the Program beneficiaries were appropriately cared for and satisfied with the benefits they received. Data show that there were 4.13 million households and 5.19 million people receiving five-guarantee benefits in rural areas across the country in 1958.[11]

Some communities started to run pilot nursing homes for the old people who had nobody to take care of them. In early 1956, Xinghua Town of Baiquan County in Heilongjiang Province opened a nursing home to look after 11 old people. Thereafter, two types of care emerged under the Five-Guarantee Program for elderly people: one was living in nursing homes and the other was staying at their own homes to receive support from local communities. In December 1958, the Sixth Plenary Session of the Eighth Central Committee of the Communist Party of China passed the *Resolution on Several Issues Concerning People's Communes*, which pointed out that "it is necessary to open nursing homes and provide a living place for the old people who don't have anyone to take care of them." After that, nursing homes sprang up all over the country. Data show that there were 150,000 nursing homes in China at the end of 1958, supporting more than 3 million old people.[12]

Due to the influence of "leftist" ideology, the Five-Guarantee Program encountered difficult challenges in its development. During the Great Leap Forward, many local governments disregarded the needs and economic resources of rural cooperatives and communes which, in addition to supporting the nursing homes, were also required to provide free food and grains for five-guarantee beneficiaries who stayed at their own homes and to ensure their living standards the same as other cooperative or commune members. Large-scale nursing homes sprang up everywhere across the country in a short

10 Local History Compilation Committee of Anhui Province, ed. 1992. *Chronicle of Anhui Province: Civil Administration*. Anhui People's Publishing House. 237.

11 Editorial Office of *Series on Contemporary China*, ed. 1994. *Civil Administration in Contemporary China* (Volume 2). Contemporary China Publishing House. 105–106.

12 Editorial Office of *Series on Contemporary China*, ed. 1994. *Civil Administration in Contemporary China* (Volume 2). Contemporary China Publishing House. 105–106.

time. In just one year, Fujian Province opened 1,160 nursing homes and orphanages, supporting 21,619 old people and orphans.[13] At the end of 1958, the 9,786 nursing homes in Anhui Province had 174,896 residents, accounting for 48.4 percent of the total number of people eligible for the Program, which stood at 361,017. A nursing home resident typically received items worth 80 to 100 yuan per year, including 250 or 300 kilo raw grains, a ration of cooking oil that was the same or slightly higher than the level for ordinary commune members, and a specified number of cloth vouchers.[14] During the difficult three years in wake of the Great Leap Forward, many communes and production brigades had to close their nursing homes due to the lack of food and financial resources, and most of the people living in those facilities returned to their production brigades. Data show that in 1962, there were only 30,000 nursing homes in the country, with only 550,000 residents, an 80 percent decline from the number in 1958.[15] In 1962, there were only 89 nursing homes in 28 counties in Fujian Province, with 1,457 residents. The number of five-guarantee beneficiaries outside nursing homes dropped to 40,000, and the benefits provided by the Program were limited to grains and meals money or grains only.[16] There were only 2,684 nursing homes in Anhui Province, with 50,991 residents, accounting for 12.8 percent of the total number of five-guarantee beneficiaries in the province.[17]

After 1962, local governments took various measures to adjust and improve the Program. They rolled out policies regarding the provision of support for the most vulnerable groups in rural areas by the people's communes in accordance with the *Amendment to the Regulations of Rural People's Communes (Draft)*, strengthened the supervision at local levels, and made overall arrangements to better support the Program's target groups and other vulnerable groups. For example, in 1962, the Civil Affairs Department of Guangxi Zhuang Autonomous Region formulated the *Provisional Measures for Offering Subsidies by the People's Communes to Five-guarantee Beneficiaries and Other Vulnerable Groups (Draft)*. According to the *Amendment to the Regulations*

13 Local History Compilation Committee of Fujian Province, ed. 1997. *Chronicle of Fujian Province: Civil Administration*. Fangzhi Publishing House. 104.

14 Local History Compilation Committee of Anhui Province, ed. 1992. *Chronicle of Anhui Province: Civil Administration*. Anhui People's Publishing House. 238.

15 Editorial Office of *Series on Contemporary China*, ed. 1994. *Civil Administration in Contemporary China* (Volume 2), Contemporary China Publishing House. 107.

16 Local History Compilation Committee of Fujian Province, ed. 1997. *Chronicle of Fujian Province: Civil Administration*. Fangzhi Publishing House. 104.

17 Local History Compilation Committee of Anhui Province, ed. 1992. *Chronicle of Anhui Province: Civil Administration*. Anhui People's Publishing House. 238.

of Rural People's Communes (Draft), Jilin Province set aside three to five percent of the commune's distributable income as public welfare fund to support five-guarantee beneficiaries and other vulnerable groups. In March 1964, the *Measures of Offering Subsidies for Five-guarantee Beneficiaries and Other Disadvantaged Groups in the People's Communes in Rural Areas of Jilin Province* was issued, setting up the standards and forms of subsidies for the target groups.[18]

During the "Cultural Revolution", the Program was neglected and even abandoned in some places. Some officials at the basic-level of administration turned a blind eye to the difficulties of the target groups. Despite the policy that "everyone eats from the same big pot" (*da guo fan*), some of the target groups had limited access to adequate staple food, lived in dilapidated houses, and wore shabby clothes. A survey shows that there were 23 five-guarantee households in Liangxiang Commune of Fangshan County, Beijing in the winter of 1978 and 9 of them lived in dilapidated houses, accounting for 40 percent of the total number of households receiving benefits under the Program in Liangxiang Commune. Among the target groups, four households lived in loaned private houses, two in pig farms, two in guardrooms, and one in breeding rooms. The number of nursing homes nationwide dropped significantly. By the end of 1978, there were only 7,175 nursing homes, with over 100,000 residents, and the living conditions were very poor. Some nursing homes became workshops or drop-in centers and the wellbeing of the residents was not guaranteed. These problems had a very bad effect in the society and seriously undermined the Program.[19]

Despite the many setbacks and problems of the Program during the time period of planned economy, the establishment of this rural social security system after the founding of the People's Republic of China nonetheless played an important role in providing the most needed support for the most vulnerable and disadvantaged groups who would have otherwise lived in miserable conditions. The Program brought obvious benefits to the society in consolidating the victory of the Chinese Revolution, supporting the recovery and development of national economy and promoting Chinese traditional virtues of respecting the elderly, caring for the young and helping the poor. It reflected the superiority of the socialist system and promoted social stability. Under the leadership of the CPC and the Chinese government and with the support of the rural

18 Local History Compilation Committee of Jilin Province, ed. 1991. *Chronicle of Jilin Province: Politics (Civil Administration)*. Jilin People's Publishing House. 209.

19 Editorial Office of *Series on Contemporary China*, ed. 1994. *Civil Administration in Contemporary China* (Volume 2). Contemporary China Publishing House. 107.

collective economy, the Program made history by providing support for more than 2.5 million five-guarantee households.

2 Elderly Care Facilities Co-financed by Towns and Villages during the Market-Oriented Reforms (1979–2001)

Since the economic reforms, most of rural China adopted the household contract responsibility system. This resulted, on the one hand, in rapid growth in the rural economy and substantial improvement in farmers' income and lives. On the other hand, with the transformation of rural production management and distribution models, village-level collective organizations did not have adequate funds to meet the growing needs for public welfare, and some rural collective economic organizations were dissolved. In addition, regional imbalance in economic development became increasingly prominent, and the Five-Guarantee Program previously implemented by production teams and brigades under the collective economy could not afford to provide the support for the target groups, leading to significant drop of their living standards.

To better understand the living conditions of the target groups, learn from the past, and improve the operational efficiency of the Program, the Ministry of Civil Affairs conducted the first national survey of the Program's target groups from the end of 1982 through the beginning of 1984. The survey achieved many purposes. First, it allowed relevant authorities to get a clear understanding of the numbers of eligible persons and the forms and standards of support. By the end of 1983, there were more than 2.526 million rural households, or over 2.9501 million persons eligible for the Program, including 2.612 million old people, 223,500 people with disabilities, and 114,600 orphans, accounting respectively for 88.54 percent, 7.58 percent, and 3.88 percent of the total number of five-guarantee beneficiaries. According to the survey, more than 2.8378 million people received benefits, accounting for 96.18 percent of the target population. Among the population that received benefits under the Program, more than 169,400 people received support from nursing homes, accounting for 5.74 percent; more than 2.4114 million people were provided for by rural collectives, accounting for 81.73 percent; more than 257,000 people were provided for by relatives, friends and neighbors, accounting for 8.71 percent. In addition, more than 165,100 people received a fixed amount of allowances regularly from the state.

Second, the survey facilitated the implementation of the Program. During the survey, errors and flaws of the Program were corrected. Nearly 300,000 eligible but previously not supported people were now included in the Program. The newly added beneficiaries in Beijing, Hebei, Shandong, Guangdong and other provinces and cities accounted for more than 30 percent of the total number prior to the survey. Many local authorities adjusted the levels of benefits. There were 180,000 people receiving five-guarantee benefits in Shandong Province. The ration of food each beneficiary received increased by 17 kilograms per year and their allowances each increased by 27 yuan per year. According to the statistics of 13 provinces including Shanxi, Anhui and Hubei, 37,000 homes were built or renovated, more than 45,000 pieces of clothing, more than 1.7 million kilograms of food, and more than 800,000 yuan in cash were provided to the target population, while caregivers were assigned to 590,000 people who were incapable of independent living. During the survey, many local CPC or government officials attached great importance to the Five-Guarantee Program and actively helped the target groups solve their problems. Many local political and social groups, including the militia organizations and the All-China Women's Federation offices encouraged their members to pair with the Program's beneficiaries to help them with daily activities, such as fetching water and firewood, cooking, doing laundry, and seeking medical treatment.

Third, the survey promoted the development of nursing homes. During the survey, 3,461 nursing homes were built nationwide and the number of residents rose by more than 31,800, an increase of 33 percent and 23 percent, respectively. Many nursing homes were renovated or expanded to improve the living conditions for the residents and ensure that they could spend their twilight years in peace.[20]

Fourth, relevant rules and regulations were formulated. Based on the survey results, local authorities summarized their past experience, and rolled out measures and regulations in accordance to local conditions. For example, the *Interim Measures for the Provision of Five-guarantee Benefits* issued by the People's Government of Hebei Province in 1983 set out regulations on matters such as eligibility, supporting methods, property disposal, establishing nursing homes, and appraisal of organization and management.

The survey revealed the following major problems. First, benefits were not fully provided. In some rural communities, beneficiaries could receive only one or two (rather than five) kinds of benefits, and some of them could only obtain grains. Some local authorities would specify the contribution of each household to the Program, and then ask the beneficiaries to collect grain and cash themselves from those households. Sometimes, they asked the beneficiaries

20 Editorial Office of *Series on Contemporary China*, ed. 1994. *Civil Administration in Contemporary China* (Volume 2). Contemporary China Publishing House. 109–110.

to go and eat at the households by turns, or assigned the farm fields to the beneficiaries for self-support. In some provinces, 27 percent of the target beneficiaries supported themselves through farming on assigned fields or farming for others. In some areas, the figure reached 50 percent.

Second, the level of support was low. The benefits provided to some beneficiaries were inadequate to meet their basic needs. In some areas, the grain ration for the target groups was only about 100 kilograms per year. The target groups had to collect firewood by themselves. When they fell sick, there was nobody around to take care of them. They lived in dilapidated houses with lots of difficulties.

Third, household contributions to the Program were uneven. There were huge regional gaps in the development of rural collective economy in China. Border regions and mountainous and remote areas had long suffered poverty with low average income, and they had large numbers of the target population. It was very difficult for people to contribute to the Program when they had financial difficulty themselves. For example, a village of Chengguan town in Jingxing county, Hebei province had only 20 households, 7 of whom were eligible for receiving benefits of the Program. That means less than two households had to support one five-guarantee household. The burden was indeed too heavy.[21]

In response to the problems of the Program and the changes in rural social and economic system, the Fourth Plenary Session of the 11th CPC Central Committee adopted the *Decision of the CPC Central Committee on Several Issues Concerning Accelerating Agricultural Development* in September 1979, which pointed out that "collective welfare programs must be improved along with the development of collective economy, to ensure better aid to old people, orphans, people with disabilities, disabled veterans, families of dead soldiers, and other disadvantaged and vulnerable groups."[22] The CPC Central Committee issued in September 1980 the *Notice on Further Strengthening and Improving the Agricultural Production Responsibility System* and emphasized that the communes and production teams with the practice of household responsibility system should have proper measures in place to aid the families of dead soldiers, the five-guarantee households, and other disadvantaged and vulnerable groups."[23] The

21 Editorial Office of *Series on Contemporary China*, ed. 1994. *Civil Administration in Contemporary China* (Volume 2). Contemporary China Publishing House. 112–113.

22 Party Literature Research Office of the CPC Central Committee, ed. 1992. *A Collection of Important Documents on Government Work Relating to Agriculture and the Countryside in the New Era*. Central Party Literature Press. 33.

23 Party Literature Research Office of the CPC Central Committee, ed. 1992. *A Collection of Important Documents on Government Work Relating to Agriculture and the Countryside in the New Era*. Central Party Literature Press. 61.

CPC Central Committee in January 1982 approved and forwarded the *Minutes of the National Rural Work Conference*, which pointed out that "Rural collectives must set up reserve funds to aid families of dead soldiers, the five-guarantee households, and other disadvantaged and vulnerable groups." Local authorities were required to step up support for target populations. In order to ensure reliable sources of funding for the Program, the CPC Central Committee and the State Council issued the *Notice on Stopping Noncompliance in Fund Transfer and Collection in Rural Areas* in October 1985, specifying that "Money used by towns and villages ... to fund the Program and other social security matters should in principle come from taxes and other charges required by law. Before the establishment of this system ... the primary source of funding for social security programs is public service taxes."[24] The *Regulations on Farmers' Taxes and Agricultural Labor Management* promulgated by the State Council in December 1991 also stipulated: "Village deductions should include a provident fund, a public welfare fund, and a management fund", of which "the public welfare fund should be used to finance the Five-guarantee Program, subsidize households of extreme difficulty, pay for the costs of Cooperative Medical Care, and other social security matters." "Town fees can be used to finance the Five-guarantee Program. If town fees were used for the Program, no expenditure should be duplicated in village deductions."[25] The aforementioned decisions, notices, and regulations of the CPC Central Committee and the State Council, as well as local practices, helped the Program shifting from policy to legal framework and laid the foundation for a legal framework of the Program. They provided the foundation for the Program to transit from previously operated by production teams and brigades and financed by the public welfare fund during the people's commune era to now operated primarily by the town government with village deductions and town fees as the main source of funding.

In January 1994, the State Council promulgated the *Regulations on the Rural Five-Guarantee Program*, the first ever regulatory document specifically concerning the Program. It marked the start of a process towards standardized and law-based operation of the Program. Moreover, it showed the significant institutional changes of the Program in the context of market-oriented reforms. First, the eligibility criteria for five-guarantee beneficiaries were legally established. In the past, the definition of five-guarantee beneficiaries had been vague in policy documents, which generally included widows, orphans, senior

24 Party Literature Research Office of the CPC Central Committee, ed. 1992. *A Collection of Important Documents on Government Work Relating to Agriculture and the Countryside in the New Era*. Central Party Literature Press. 355.

25 *The People's Daily*, December 13, 1991. 2.

residents, disabled persons and members who had no work capability and no providers.[26] The 1994 *Regulations* stipulate that the Program shall cover only the seniors, the minors and the disabled who had no legal providers or if their legal providers were unable to support them, and who were unable to work and had no source of living.[27] Only those who met all of the above three criteria were eligible for five-guarantee benefits.

Second, both the scale and scope of the benefits improved. The benefits offered by the Program during the people's commune era were food, clothing, fuel/firewood, burial services, and education at the average level of income and resources distribution of the collectives. After the economic reforms, the Program benefits changed to better support the target groups, which included food, clothing, housing, health care, and burial services (or education for minors). The standards of support were designed to ensure the living standard of the target groups the same as the average fellow villagers. Data show that the average amount of money paid by the Program was 670 yuan per capita and 1,070 yuan for each nursing home resident in 1994, exceeding the national average income in 1993. The benefits received by most of the target population were enough to help them meet their basic needs.[28]

Third, sources of funding for the Program became more reliable. In the past, the Program had been mainly financed by the public welfare fund of the production teams and brigades. After the economic reforms, the sources of funding began to diversify, including village deductions, town fees, support of relatives, and support of other persons who, in return, were allowed to cultivate the beneficiaries' farmland. Among them, the town fees were a more reliable source of funding. Since 1985, this financing model had been promoted nationwide. In the meantime, burgeoning town – and village-owned enterprises became an additional source of funding. In 1994, 31,000 towns, 65 percent of all towns across the country, collected public services fees, and 853.72 million yuan was used to aid the 1.39 million five-guarantee beneficiaries not living in nursing homes, accounting for more than 62 percent of the persons supported by the Program in a decentralized manner. At the same time, the state also increased the effort to support the Program. In addition to unscheduled aid, it promoted a regularized aid mechanism on a national scale, requiring local authorities to give priority to the target population when distributing relief

26 *The People's Daily*, January 28, 1994. 3.

27 *The People's Daily*, January 28, 1994. 3.

28 Party Literature Research Office of the CPC Central Committee, ed. 1991. *Manuscripts by Mao Zedong after the Founding of the People's Republic* (Volume 5). Central Party Literature Press. 199–200.

funds and supplies. In 1994, the country allocated 75.54 million yuan in relief to the five-guarantee beneficiaries, accounting for 27.8 percent of the country's total rural social relief expenditures.[29]

Fourth, the promulgation of the *Interim Measures for the Management of Rural Nursing Homes* in March 1997 regularized the construction, management and operation of rural nursing homes, and provided the policy guidance for their development.

After the *Regulations* (1994) and the *Interim Measures* (1997) were issued, local authorities stepped up their efforts to establish relevant rules and regulations for the implementation of the programs. All provinces, autonomous regions and municipalities formulated detailed rules, in light of local realities, for the implementation of the Five-Guarantee Program and the management of nursing homes. Counties, cities, and districts with agricultural population set up measures on the implementation of the Program and the management of nursing homes. Most town governments and nursing homes formulated their policy documents. These regulations and policies at central, provincial and local levels helped form a coordinated unified system. It not only laid a solid foundation for the institutionalization and standardization of the Five-Guarantee Program, but also made the Program the most complete and efficient primary work in rural social security in China.

In summary, the Five-Guarantee Program was well implemented in most areas to ensure the basic needs for the target groups during the economic reforms. The Program also facilitated family planning in rural areas. When people witnessed that old people without family providers could still enjoy their twilight years peacefully with a life even better than those with children, many people no longer adhered to the old ideas that they must have children so that they could be taken care of in their old age or have a son to carry on the family. They began to actively comply with the family planning policy. According to the data published in the *Statistical Bulletin of the Ministry of Civil Affairs on the Development of Civil Affairs* (2000), the Program was well implemented in rural areas in 2000 and "the five-guarantee households who were aided by the collectives reached 2.081 million, an increase of 6.5 percent over the previous year, and the money spent by the collectives on the Program was 2.05 billion yuan, an increase of 1.5 percent over the previous year."[30]

---

29 Party Literature Research Office of the CPC Central Committee, ed. 1991. *Manuscripts by Mao Zedong after the Founding of the People's Republic* (Volume 5). Central Party Literature Press. 209.

30 http://www.mca.gov.cn/articaJ/content/WJYL-ZH/200482082342.html.

3 Establishment of a Modern Social Security System in the New Socialist Countryside with Government Funds as the Primary and the Collective Funds, Land Revenue and Social Assistance as the Secondary Sources (2002 to Present)

The continuing market-oriented reform and the rural tax reform since the mid-1990s has led to continuous development of the rural economy, reduced farmers' burdens and increased their incomes. In the meantime, rural Five-Guarantee Program has encountered many new realities and problems. In the early stage of the tax reform, the primary funding sources for the Program changed from "village deductions or town fees" to agricultural taxes and surcharges. After further tax reforms and the abolition of agricultural taxes and surcharges, the Program was funded primarily by payments transferred from higher-level governments and from the budgets of various local governments. In theory, the change should have a positive impact on the life of the target groups. However, according to a nationwide survey conducted by the Ministry of Civil Affairs from August to October 2003, the change did not bring about better protection for them. There were many problems.

First, a major problem was the failure to cover a significant portion of the target population. According to the data provided by the Department of Disaster Relief and Social Assistance of the Ministry of Civil Affairs, as of the end of 2002, only 2,968,200 people in rural areas had been aided by the Scheme, accounting for about 52.04 percent of the target population. That means, nearly half of the target population were not covered.[31] In poor villages, it was even more difficult to implement the Program when ordinary farmers still lived a hard life.

Second, the standards of support were difficult to be sustained. According to relevant regulations, the Program should ensure the target groups a living standard no less than that of the average villagers. However, that became hardly possible in some places when a huge gap existed between the announced standard of cash assistance and the actual living allowances received by the target groups. According to the data provided by the Department of Disaster Relief and Social Assistance of the Ministry of Civil Affairs, the standard support for those in nursing homes fell from 2,173 yuan in 2001 to 1,691 yuan in 2002, and

---

31 Hong Dayong et al. 2004. "Dilemma and Way Out: A Study of the Rural Five-Guarantee Scheme in the Post-Collective Era." *Journal of Renmin University of China*, (1).

the standard support for those living at home fell from 1,262 yuan to 958 yuan, a decrease of 22.2 percent and 24.1 percent respectively.[32]

Third, it was difficult to have all the five types of benefits delivered. Survey results showed that except for the burial services, many local authorities had some difficulties in providing all the other benefits. In some areas, the five types of benefits were reduced to two types (food and burial services) or even one type (food). As for housing, the target groups always had the worse in rural areas if they did not have external assistance and help. Access to health care remained the biggest challenge in the delivery of the five-guarantee benefits. The target groups had no sure access to primary healthcare whether they lived in nursing homes or at their own homes. Even in towns and villages with best conditions, the target groups only received healthcare reimbursement up to 200–300 yuan each person per year, which was too little for those who were feeble and old.

Fourth, daily care for the target groups was neglected. The survey shows that a large percentage of the five-guarantee beneficiaries were semi-dependent or completely dependent old people who needed assistance in their daily life. While those living in nursing homes might receive care from staff members or fellow residents, daily care for those living at their own homes was mostly neglected.

The causes for these problems were often complicated, but the following were particularly noteworthy. First, the target population increased rapidly, which was caused by changes in rural demographic structure with the increase of life expectancy and rapid growth of older population, and prior deliberate underreporting. Moreover, people who were identified as the "three withouts" (without sources of income, work capability, and legal supporters or supporters unable to work) had previously relied on farming to support themselves, but now they became old and eligible for the Five-Guarantee Program. Some old people who used to rely on the support of their relatives and friends to cultivate their land also became eligible for the Program because they lost the sources of support when their relatives were increasingly unwilling to farm their land and be their providers due to very low income from farming and increased financial burdens.

Second, the funding of the Program was not guaranteed. Shortage of funds was one of the major challenges in the implementation of the Program. Before the tax reforms, major sources of funding came from village deductions and town fees ("*santi wutong*"). Although many local authorities failed to collect

32 Gu Xin and Jiang Wei. 2004. "Tax Reform and the Institutionalization of the Rural Five-Guarantee Scheme Financing System." *Jiangsu Social Sciences*, (3).

the levies in full, the funds were able to meet the funding need due to broad sources. After the tax reforms, the funding of the Program came from revenues collected from agricultural tax surcharges (20 percent of the agriculture taxes). Revenues thus collected were also used to pay wages and office expenses of village-level organizations. However, the revenues were generally much less than the those from the village and town levies before the reforms, and in many areas, they were not even enough to cover the expenses of one type of benefits under the Program. Transfer payments from higher-level governments were of general budget support and the money for the Five-Guarantee Program was often taken to fund other programs in the process of transfer from the provincial to county to town levels when there were not enough funds for all programs. The Five-Guarantee Program was most likely to be eroded and neglected, making it difficult for the transfer payments from higher-level governments to reach the target groups. Moreover, many town governments faced serious fiscal stresses as debts of local governments became a nationwide problem. Under such circumstances, it was indeed very difficult to count on the town governments to guarantee the funding of the Program.

Third, the Five-Guarantee Program did not adjust timely to the changes in society. The underlying cause of funding shortage was the institutional constraints. The *Regulations on Rural Five-Guarantee Program* promulgated by the State Council in 1994 was essentially a continuation of the model adopted during the planned economy under which the collectives were the main entities responsible for aiding the target groups. Because it did not take into consideration the social and economic changes in rural areas, the Program became incompatible with the above-mentioned rural tax reforms and the current public finance system. The purpose of public finance is not for profitable financial gains but to finance public administration and social welfare programs. The Five-Guarantee Program is not a collective welfare program but a social security program with specific target groups. It is against the essential elements of social security and the purpose of public finance to hold farmers and rural collective organizations responsible for financing a social security program.[33]

Fourth, the development of rural communities lagged behind and the level of community services was low. The Program is not merely about subsidizing low-incomers. It has the two components of subsidizing the income and providing services. In the era of collective economy, collective organizations were able to perform both, allowing the Program to be effectively implemented.

33 Ye Xingqing and Zhang Shunxi. 2003. "The Rural Five-Guarantee Scheme Urgently Needs Reform." *China Social Welfare*, (12).

However, with the changes in market-oriented reforms, the Program increasingly focused on subsidizing the income and neglecting the daily care of the target groups, with the needs of many old people severely marginalized and the Program greatly weakened. So far, China's community development effort has been focused on cities. There is an urgent need for developing rural communities and improving their services, which is an important part of the initiatives of building a new socialist countryside.

On March 1, 2006, a revised *Regulations on the Rural Five-Guarantee Program* (hereafter referred to as the "New Regulations") came into effect. The New Regulations was based on the practices of past 50 years and the results of studies on the current rural economic and social situations, especially the situation after rural tax reforms. With the introduction of the New Regulations, the Program becomes primarily state-funded. It not only deals with the immediate needs of five-guarantee households, but also intends as a long-term mechanism to meet their basic needs. Compared with the 1994 Regulations (hereinafter referred to as the "Old Regulations"), the new version has established an improved and more comprehensive system that includes more feasible measures. The significance of the New Regulations can be summarized as follows:

1. The New Regulations accomplished the historic transition of the Program from a farmer mutual assistance model to a modern social security program with the state as its primary source of funding and collective funds, land revenue and social assistance as its secondary sources of funding. The Old Regulations defined the Program as a rural collective welfare program financed by village deductions and town fees. The New Regulations stipulates that the Program is primarily financed by the government, with local governments allocating budget for the Program and the central government providing financial support to local governments when necessary. At the same time, it attaches importance to the auxiliary role of collective funds and land revenue. In rural areas that have profit-making collective businesses, part of their income may be set aside to help finance the Program. Those people of target groups who entrust their farmland to others for cultivation via contract should keep their income.
2. The New Regulations provides for a natural growth in five-guarantee benefits, enabling the Program's target groups to benefit from the reform and development as well. According to the Old Regulations, the standards should in principle be determined by the town government, which is not conducive to the implementation of relevant policies and balancing out the different development of regions. The New Regulations requires higher-level administrative bodies to formulate the standards

for benefits. These can be provincial governments, or governments of cities (those with subsidiary districts) and counties, provided they file with the provincial government. It is also stipulated that the benefits should be timely adjusted according to the improvement of the average living standards of local villagers to ensure a natural growth of benefits.

3. The New Regulations strengthens the establishment and management of rural care service facilities of the Program. The Old Regulations required the town governments to build nursing homes when conditions permit but did not specify the provisions of staffing and financing. The New Regulations stipulates that people's governments at all levels should incorporate the establishment of care service facilities into the economic and social development plan, and that county and town governments should provide necessary equipment, funds, and adequately trained staff for such facilities.
4. The New Regulations sets up supervision and management rules in relation to the Program. It stipulates the responsibilities of the departments of civil affairs, finance, and auditing at all levels and the town governments in supervision of the management of the Program. It establishes a public announcement system to ensure public oversight. It also stipulates that relevant agencies should comply with the measures of national security, fire control, sanitation, accounting, and other regulations. The New Regulations contains a new chapter on legal liabilities for the administrative staff, care service providers, and members of village committees to enhance the accountability for any violations.[34]

Statistics show that the Program now covers 3.285 million people, providing them with support that is equivalent to 989 yuan per capita annually, which meets their basic needs relatively well. Among the beneficiaries, 632,000 people live in over 30,000 nursing homes across the country. In economically developed areas such as Shanghai, Beijing, Guangdong, Jiangsu, and Zhejiang, the standard of support has reached 60 percent to 70 percent of local farmers' average net income. In many places, the Program helps the guarantee recipients with a decent and comfortable living. Many old people eligible for the five-guarantee benefits enjoy their twilight years in nursing homes, and some of them happily married there.[35] In the past 50 years, the Program has played an important role in promoting the economy and stabilizing social order in

34 *In-depth Implementation of the Regulations on the Rural Five-Guarantee Scheme and Initiation of a New Phase in the Promotion of the Scheme*, http://www.societynews.cn/zgshb/ShowArticle.asp?ArticleID=282.

35 *The China Youth Daily*, March 2, 2006.

rural areas, and shaping up a good image of the CPC and the Chinese government to reflect the superiority of the socialist system.

The evolution of the Program over the years is a process of change and adaptation, particularly in the context of the ongoing rural economic reforms and social changes in China. We may roughly divide the process into three stages:

1. During the first stage (from 1956 to 1978), the Program, which was launched in the 1950s during the agricultural cooperative movement, was a collectively financed program operated by production teams and brigades, relying on their public welfare fund for financial support. At the time, China prioritized the development of heavy industries and thus did not have enough resources to aid farmers and support the development of rural areas and agriculture. The country had to rely on rural collective organizations to meet the basic needs of the disadvantaged and vulnerable groups. Under the people's commune system, the main entities responsible for implementing the Program were production teams and brigades, and the primary source of funding was their collective public welfare funds.
2. During the second stage (from 1979 to 2001), the Program remained collectively financed, though with village deductions and town fees as the primary sources of funding. This model was adopted for the purpose of adapting to the market-oriented reforms of rural economy. After the adoption of the household responsibility system, collective economic organizations in most rural areas were no longer responsible for organizing agricultural production activities. The farmer's family became the unit to engage in productive activities and control the income. Public funds of the collective organizations decreased significantly, and some collectives were dismantled. As a result, social security and welfare programs that had previously relied on collective resources were now seriously underfunded. In addition, after China began to implement the economic reforms and opening up policy, regional gaps in socioeconomic development and the target population, along with uneven burdens of social security on farmers, were important factors that led to the reform of the Program. The transition to a new model was the promulgation of the *Regulations on the Rural Five-Guarantee Program (1994)*, which specified town governments as the main entities responsible for operating and managing the Program, while village deductions and town fees were the primary sources of funds.
3. During the third stage (from 2002 to present), the Program has become a modern social security program that relies on government funding, and complemented by collective funds, land revenue and social assistance.

This model is not only a product of China's efforts to deepen the market-oriented economic reform, but also a necessary part of a modern rural social security system. At present, China is in the middle of industrialization, a stage where industries begin to play a role in supporting the development of agriculture. With the country growing stronger, the government has the financial resources needed for the Program. Therefore, the New Regulations in 2006 stipulates that the primary source of funding will be transfer payments from higher-level governments and allocations in the budget of local governments. It can be said that the promulgation of the New Regulations is an important sign that the new model has basically taken shape.

In summary, the changes that occurred in these stages are a process of institutionalization, standardization, legislation and improvement of the Program benefits. It is a transition from farmers' mutual assistance and self-financing to a public financed model in the exploration of establishing a modern rural social security system in China.

CHAPTER 3

Building and Reforming China's Rural Social Security System: a 60-Year Review

Chen Shaohui, Li Liqin and Zheng Xiaoling *

Abstract

In the early years of the People's Republic of China, while providing relatively complete social insurance programs for employees in cities, the government established a social security system in rural areas based on collective economy and featuring collective security. Since then, the rural social security system in China has shown the characteristic of path dependency in the process of change. After sixty years of efforts to build and reform its rural social security system, China has gradually put in place a social security system that is independent from the "production system" and towards a uniform social security model in urban and rural areas.

Keywords

rural social security system – progressive reform – path dependency – institutional changes

As the issues of agriculture, rural communities and farmers draw more attention nationwide and the Chinese government increases its support for the development of rural areas, the rural social security system has become a hot research topic in the academic world. It is worth noting, however, that the existing research is more about historical facts and lacks theoretical analysis. It is even rare to see the examination of historical changes in China's rural social security system from the perspective of economic history. The introduction of

* Chen Shaohui, professor at the School of Economics, Fujian Normal University; Li Liqin, MA student, program in Labor and Social Security at the School of Public Administration, Fujian Normal University; Zheng Xiaoling, Ph.D. candidate in Economic History at the School of Economics, Fujian Normal University.

 | DOI:10.1163/9789004737990_004

new institutional economics provides a brand-new perspective for analyzing the institutional changes of rural social security. From the angle of path dependency, this paper looks at the evolution of China's rural social security system over the past six decades and its future projection.

1 Rural Social Security Based on Collective Economy: from 1949 to 1977

In the early years of the People's Republic of China (PRC), while providing urban employees with sound social insurance programs, the Chinese government introduced collective security based on collective economy for rural residents. Under the rural collective security system, the earnings of rural communes, featuring collective labor, collective accounting and unified allocation, were used to meet the basic needs of rural residents. It mainly comprised the Five-Guarantee System, the disaster relief and support system, and the cooperative medical care system.

1.1 *Rural Five-Guarantee System*

The Five-Guarantee System (FGS) in rural China was established in the period of agricultural cooperation. In 1956, the idea of "Five Guarantees" was put forth in the Standard Charter of Advanced Agricultural Cooperatives for the purpose of providing assistance to members of the cooperatives who were elderly, widowed or disabled.[1] The National Outline for Agricultural Development, adopted in 1960, further specified that agricultural cooperatives should provide "food, clothing, fuel, education (for children and juveniles) and burial expenses" for widowers who had no help.[2] Later on, housing and medical care support was added to ensure the living standard of those people not below the local average. People covered by the FGS were supported by designated service providers or villagers' committees. During the Great Leap Forward in 1958, the number of rural homes for the elderly grew to 150,000, with more than three million elderly people taken care of.[3]

---

1 Party Literature Research Office of the CPC Central Committee, ed. 1994. *Selected Important Documents Since the Founding of the People's Republic of China* (Volume 8). Beijing: Central Party Literature Publishing House. 364.

2 Editorial Committee of *An Overview of China's Social Security System*, ed. 1995. *An Overview of China's Social Security System*. Beijing: China Democracy and Legal Publishing House. 943.

3 Policy Research Office of the Ministry of Civil Affairs. 1997. *Social Security in Rural China*. Beijing: China Social Publishing House. 71.

1.2 *Rural Disaster Relief and Support System*

The rural disaster relief and support system was that in the event of natural disasters, the government would provide the funds and supplies to meet the basic needs of rural residents for food, clothing, housing, medical care, etc. Following the founding of the PRC, the Chinese government paid great attention to disaster preparedness and relief. It established a relatively comprehensive disaster relief and support system in rural areas, combining both programs of regular and temporary support. From 1958 to 1978, the government allocated RMB 9.45 billion in relief funds to support the affected rural residents, which helped maintain rural social stability despite the shortages of materials.[4]

1.3 *Rural Cooperative Medical Care System*

Cooperative medical care, a basic component of China's rural healthcare system, was to provide rural community members with basic healthcare services with government support at all levels in the principle of mutual assistance among participants. With the development of people's communes, the cooperative medical care system had grown to cover ninety percent of all rural residents across the country by the mid-1970s.[5] Cooperative medical care, the health clinics of agricultural cooperatives, and the large numbers of barefoot doctors helped overcome the shortages of medical services and medicines in the vast rural China. It was considered by the WHO as a successful example of developing rural healthcare in developing countries.

During the planned economy period, China established a rural social security system that was based on collective economy and characterized by collective security. The social security system in this period supported the strategy of giving priority to industrialization, ensured meeting the basic needs of the rural population, and maintained the stability of rural society when the level of economic development was low and social security needs were high. It also showed the characteristic of path dependency in its reform process.

2 Rural Social Security System within the "Production System": from 1978 to the Mid-1980s

After the Third Plenary Session of the Eleventh CPC Central Committee in 1978, farmers obtained the use right of contracted land, while the collective security

4 Policy Research Office of the Ministry of Civil Affairs. 1997. *Social Security in Rural China*. Beijing: China Social Publishing House. 71.

5 Dong Keyong. 2008. *30 Years of China's Economic Reform: Social Security (1978–2008)*. Chongqing: Chongqing University Press. 152.

based on the people's commune system gradually lost its solid organizational support and economic foundation. Therefore, the rural security system had to return to the path of leveraging family support. In this period, while the rural collective security system was disintegrating, an alternative social security system was not yet put into place for the farmers. Instead, land was used as both the means of production and social security.

2.1 *The Decline of Rural Collective Security after the Disintegration of People's Commune System*

The introduction of contracted land use led to the decline and collapse of rural collective economy. As a result, the FGS and cooperative medical care system were gradually weakened to the point of disintegration. As the collective economic base was seriously weakened, the life and old-age support of many people covered by the FGS were seriously affected in the areas where the basic living allowances were not secured. Rural cooperative medical care also suffered a significant decline due to lack of funding. According to a survey conducted in 1985, the number of administrative villages practicing cooperative medical care dropped sharply from ninety percent in the mid-1970s to five percent. In 1989, only 4.8 percent of the administrative villages in the country were still offering cooperative medical care.[6] Except for a few developed suburban villages, most farmers had to return to traditional family support as a source of security.

2.2 *The Overlap of Rural Social Security System and Social Production System*

Since the economic reforms and opening up, family and land have once again become the main source of social security for rural residents. Rural social security system and rural social production system overlapped, with the same organizational boundaries. The social security system was not separated from the social production system.

2.2.1 Family as Source of Security

The family is a basic unit of the society, consisting of members of the society because of marriage, blood ties or adoption. It is a social organization with lasting stability that allows to make flexible spending decisions. Therefore, households are the last line of defense of social security for agricultural production, which is known for its uncertainty and risks. The household contract responsibility system injected great vitality into the household economy in

6 Gu Tao and Shan Jie. 1998. "Analysis of Issues Related to the Rural Medical Insurance System and Policy Suggestions." *Chinese Health Economics*, (4).

rural areas, leading to increases in farmers' income and household savings. From 1978 to 1997, the household income of rural residents per capita increased from RMB 233 to RMB 5,940, and financial assets grew from RMB 18 to RMB 1,334 per capita. Housing conditions improved significantly. Housing area per capita increased from 8.1 square meters to 22.45 square meters. Grain stock at year end grew from sixty-four kilograms per capita in 1980 to 562 kilograms in 1997.[7] Rural households greatly enhanced the preparedness for natural disasters and the ability to deal with needs of everyday life. Family support once again became the main source of social security in rural China.

2.2.2 Land as Source of Security

After the establishment of household contract responsibility system, rural households contracted a certain amount of land and the harvest or earnings obtained from such land became the main source of income for family members to meet basic needs of life and to cope with risks associated with aging, diseases, disasters, etc. Land was once again used as both means of production and social security. Its role in providing support for rural residents can be seen in two aspects. On the one hand, the basic needs of farmers were met mainly with the income from land, which in fact made land the material base for home care or community care of elderly rural residents. On the other hand, land became the unemployment security for those farmers who left to do non-farming jobs. Some farmers would choose to go to cities to seek jobs or start business which involved risks. If they encountered risks of no jobs or business failures in cities, they could still go back and rely on the land as the last security for livelihood.

However, with industrialization and further market-oriented reforms, the risk of agricultural farming rose sharply. In the meantime, the rural social security system based on family and land was apparently weakened under the impact of institutional and social transformations. On the one hand, family support began to play a smaller role. The implementation of the family planning policy had made the size of families increasingly smaller across generations, result in the structure of 4-2-1 or 8-4-2-1. In the meantime, as people's life expectancy became longer, the proportion of middle-aged and old-age population in rural areas kept rising and the burden of caring for the old people in rural areas was also increasing. According to the census data, there were 72.85 million elderly people over the age of sixty in China, accounting for 8.2 percent of the total rural population and increasing at an annual rate

7 Duan Qinglin. 2001. "Changes in China's Rural Social Security System (1949–1999)." *Social Sciences in Ningxia* (1).

of three percent. Some demographers predict that the proportion of elderly people aged over sixty-five in China's rural areas will reach 14 to 17.7 percent in 2020, making China officially an aging society.[8] Additionally, with large-scale migration of rural surplus labor where more and more young and middle-aged rural residents leave the countryside to look for jobs elsewhere, the traditional ideas of being filial to the elderly and supporting their parents became less valued under the influence of fast changes, thus weakening the cohesion of the family. Under the combined effect of these factors, the traditional rural old-age care system featuring home care will face the challenge of short supply. On the other hand, land is losing its capacity as a means of social security. Although land is the last security for farmers, such security is declining due to the restrictions of land system and income from land. It is an indisputable fact that the cost of farming has been rising and the prices of agricultural products have been falling along with the proportion of agricultural income in recent years. Moreover, since the transfer of rural land has not resulted in a stable social security model, the land is mainly a security of employment for farmers, i.e. a security to combine one's labor with the means of production. Once the farmers lose the ability to work due to old age or other reasons, such security will be greatly weakened or even disappear.

3 Establishment of a Rural Social Security System Separated from the "Production System": from the Mid-1980s to the Present

With the overall acceleration of market-economy, industrialization and urbanization in China's rural areas, family and land are no longer able to bear the increasing social risks in rural areas (unemployment, diseases, old age, poverty, etc.). It is urgent to resolve these risks and uncertainties by establishing a modern social security system. However, because of the large population, vast areas and weak economy of rural China, it is a huge and complex project to establish a new rural social security system. It is obviously unrealistic to achieve the "full coverage" of rural residents all at once, and the government does not have the financial resources to make it happen either. Since the mid-1980s, the Chinese government started to reform the rural social security system based on family and land support while making great efforts to build an urban social security system.

8 Cheng Shaohui. 2004. "Rural Social Security: System Defects and Government Responsibility." *Journal of Fujian Normal University*, (4).

3.1 *Transforming Existing Components of Rural Social Security*

To address the absence of social security for farmers during the implementation of household contract responsibility system, China began to explore new forms of rural social security, on the basis of existing components of rural social security, to make it institutionalized, standardized and socialized.

3.1.1 Consolidating the Rural Five-Guarantee System

Because of the collapse of collective economy, people eligible for the FGS were not able to get their benefits anymore. To ensure the normal functioning of FGS, some local governments developed a new model that featured fundraising by village organizations, coordination by town organizations and care provision by family members. In 1985, town-level planning for FGS funding began to be promoted nationwide. By 1994, more than 31,000 towns across the country had carried out such overall planning, accounting for sixty-five percent of the total number of towns, making it a common source of support.[9] In January 1994, the State Council issued the *Regulations on Providing Support via the Five-Guarantee System in Rural Areas* that defined the operating procedures and contents of related work. The Regulations guided the Chinese FGS with policy and legal standards.

3.1.2 Rebuilding the Rural Cooperative Medical Care System

China has been seeking to rebuild the cooperative medical care system since the 1990s. In 1993, The CPC Central Committee issued the *Decision on Issues Concerning the Establishment of a Socialist Market Economy,* which explicitly noted the need to "develop and improve the rural cooperative medical care system." In January 1997, the CPC Central Committee and the State Council proposed to "actively and steadily develop and improve the cooperative medical care system" in the *Decision on Healthcare Reform and Development.* However, from a nationwide perspective, the efforts to rebuild the rural cooperative medical care system failed to achieve the expected results. The re-emergence of China's rural cooperative medical care began in October 2002 when the CPC Central Committee and the State Council issued the *Decision on Further Strengthening Rural Healthcare,* specifying the goal of "ensuring that the new rural cooperative medical care system cover all rural residents by 2010." In 2003, the General Office of the State Council published the Health Ministry's *Guidelines on Further Improving the Pilot Program of New Rural Cooperative Medical Care,* proposing a plan to increase government investment in the rural

9 Zheng Gongcheng. 1997. *Building a Social Security Path with Chinese Characteristics.* Wuhan: Wuhan University Press. 243.

cooperative medical care system. The 2008 *Report on the Work of the Government* further enhanced the subsidies to the cooperative medical care system to speed up the development of the new rural cooperative medical care system. As shown in Table 1, thanks to the active promotion of the central government in recent years, China's new rural cooperative medical care system has been improved in the aspects of rural coverage, level of investment and the number of beneficiaries.

TABLE 3.1 New rural cooperative medical care, 2004–2008

Year \ Item	Number of counties/districts/cities practicing new rural cooperative medical care	Coverage of rural residents (%)	Investment (in 100 million yuan)	Number of beneficiaries (in 100 million persons)
2004	333	75.2	26.37	0.76
2005	678	75.7	61.75	1.22
2006	1,451	80.7	155.81	2.72
2007	2,451	86.2	346.63	4.53
2008	2,729	91.5	662	5.85

SOURCE: MINISTRY OF HEALTH OF THE PEOPLE'S REPUBLIC OF CHINA. *SUMMARY OF CHINA'S HEALTH STATISTICS 2009*. HTTP://WWW.MOH.GOV.CN.

3.1.3 Improving the Rural Social Assistance System

The approaches to rural social assistance changed significantly after 1985, which can be seen in several aspects. Firstly, in terms of changes in disaster relief methods, paid service and free assistance were both provided to ensure meeting the basic needs of the affected people. Secondly, in terms of changes in disaster relief management, a tiered management system was adopted for relief efforts and funding in 1993. Thirdly, disaster relief was combined with poverty reduction efforts. The focus of social assistance was shifted to the eighty million poor households in the country to lift them out of poverty, especially to those in old revolutionary bases, areas of large ethnic minority populations, border and poor regions. In the 1990s, the CPC Central Committee and the State Council paid more attention to the problems of rural poverty and increased assistance to the rural poor. In 1994, a National Poverty Alleviation Plan was formulated, and a nationwide poverty alleviation campaign was carried out, mainly to support poor farmers. By the end of 1998, nearly twenty million rural residents had been lifted out of poverty, and the rural poor population was reduced to 42.1 million. About 4.4 million people in poor counties had shaken off poverty and the remaining poor population had fallen to 21.8 million.[10] In recent years, with the central government's close attention to rural poverty and the strengthening of poverty alleviation efforts, the lives of rural residents have been further improved. From 2000 to 2007, the poverty line for rural residents was raised from RMB 625 to RMB 785, while the incidence of poverty was reduced from 3.5 percent to 1.6 percent.[11]

3.2 *Introducing New Components of Rural Social Security*

In reforming traditional rural social security programs, China has sought to diversify rural social security programs in response to the shortcomings of traditional rural social security system. Some new components of rural social security have been introduced and well developed.

3.2.1 Pushing Forward the Rural Old-Age Insurance

Faced with the increasingly serious aging of rural population, China began to explore the establishment of a rural social security system in economically more developed areas since the mid-1980s, while reforming the urban social security system. In 1986, the Ministry of Civil Affairs launched a nearly five-year pilot program on the reform of rural old-age insurance. Based on that, a draft plan for rural old-age insurance system was drawn up in 1991. The *Basic Plan for County-level Old-age Social Insurance* (*trial*) was issued in January 1992, and by the end of 1997, 2008 counties and 285 prefecture-level cities had carried out related work. Moreover, more than fifty-seven percent of towns, almost all counties, nearly seventy-five percent of prefecture-level cities and eighty-seven percent of provinces had established corresponding management bodies, basically forming a network of organizations at the central, provincial, municipal, county, town and village levels.[12] As the rural old-age insurance grew, some management problems also appeared. At the end of 1997, the State Council began to look into and regulate this endeavor and found that the program was basically at a standstill. In some areas, social insurance was converted to commercial insurance, while in other areas, farmers even quitted their insurance.

---

10 Ministry of Labor and Social Security and National Bureau of Statistics. 1999. "1998 Annual Statistical Report on the Development of Labor and Social Security Programs." *China Labor and Social Security News*, June 17.

11 Ministry of Health of the People's Republic of China. "Health Statistics Yearbook of China 2008." http://www.moh.gov.cn/publicfiles/business/htmlfiles/zwgkzt/pwstj/index.htm.

12 Zhao Renwei, Lai Desheng and Wei Zhong. 2006. *China's Economic Transformation and Social Security Reform*. Beijing: Beijing Normal University Press. 134.

In sum, the exploratory efforts in those years clearly indicated the necessity of establishing a socialized rural old-age insurance system. They helped form a basic framework for China's rural old-age insurance system and gained experience in fundraising models, internal management, and external supervision, which would benefit the continuous development of old-age insurance. The pilot program on rural old-age insurance has restarted in recent years and the aim is to reach a ten percent coverage in 2009.

3.2.2 Piloting the Rural Minimum Living Needs Guarantee Program and Its Results

The Chinese government has been providing relief assistance to the rural poor for a long time, but the coverage of the assistance has been too small and the level of support too low. In addition, the limited financial resources cannot meet the basic needs of poor rural residents in some areas. In light of that, China began to explore the establishment of a rural minimum living needs guarantee program since the 1990s, on the basis of the existing FGS and disaster relief system. At the end of 1996, the Ministry of Civil Affairs officially issued the *Opinions on Accelerating the Development of Rural Social Security System* and the *Guidance for the Development of Rural Social Security System*, launching the pilot program of rural minimum living needs guarantee in the nation. From 1997, the rural minimum living needs guarantee program was gradually established in places that met the conditions. The 2007 *Report on the Work of the Government* for the first time set up the goal of "establishing a minimum living needs guarantee program to cover both urban and rural areas", thus greatly promoting the development of rural minimum living needs guarantee program. Since then, more and more poor rural families have been covered by the program, and the average allowances have been increasing (see Table 3.2).

TABLE 3.2 Minimum living needs guarantee program in rural China

	2005	2006	2007	2008	2009
People covered (in 10,000 persons)	825	1,593.9	566.3	4,305.5	4,472.7
Average allowance (yuan/person/month)			70	82.3	95.7

SOURCE: BASED ON STATISTICAL REPORTS ON THE DEVELOPMENT OF CIVIL AFFAIRS IN PREVIOUS YEARS, HTTP://WWW.MCA.GOV.CN.

3.3 *Exploring Social Security Models for Special Groups*

Along with urbanization and industrialization in China, a large number of farmers move across regions, and a large number of collectively-owned agricultural land is expropriated and converted into land for construction purposes. Inevitably a large number of migrant workers and landless farmers have emerged in this process. For these two special groups, there is currently no national arrangement for their social security, although various models have been explored and rich experience has been gained at the local level.

3.3.1 Social Security Model for Migrant Workers

All sectors of the society have reached a basic consensus on the necessity and urgency of building a social security system for migrant workers. However, in view of the structural complexity, the central government has not yet made a national plan for the social security of migrant workers. Most explorations are now made by local authorities. Local practices can be categorized into four models. The first is to directly include migrant workers in the social insurance system for urban employees. Many cities, such as Guangzhou and Shenzhen, have established social security systems for migrant workers by using this model. The second one is to reduce the participation cost for migrant workers by lowering the contribution base and contribution ratio of various social insurance items, with migrant workers receiving correspondingly lower level of social insurance benefits. This model has been adopted by many regions, such as Beijing and Zhejiang Province. The third one is the "integrated insurance model" designed specifically for migrant workers. This model was first designed and adopted by Shanghai, and a similar model was soon introduced in Chengdu. The main feature of this model is that the three insurance policies for migrant workers – work-related injury insurance, medical insurance and old-age insurance – are bundled together and the premium rate is set at a relatively low level, greatly lowering the threshold for migrant workers to participate in the insurance schemes. The fourth one is to include migrant workers in the rural social security system where they come from. Although there is not a national model of social security system for migrant workers, the various models aforementioned have achieved marked results in promoting the protection of migrant workers' rights and interests. According to the 2007 *Statistical Report on Labor and Social Security Development* jointly released by the Ministry of Human Resources and Social Security and the National Bureau of Statistics, the number of migrant workers participating in basic old-age insurance scheme was 18.46 million at the end of 2007, an increase of 4.29 million over the end of the previous year; the number of migrant workers participating in medical insurance scheme was 31.31 million, an increase of 7.64

million over the end of the previous year; the number of migrant workers participating in unemployment insurance scheme was 11.5 million; the number of migrant workers participating in work-related injury insurance scheme was 39.8 million, an increase of 14.43 million over the end of the previous year.[13]

3.3.2 Social Security Model for Landless Farmers

China has to face the difficult task, in pursuing economic growth, of settling and supporting the farmers who lose their land in the process of industrialization and urbanization. How well they are settled and supported directly relates to the progress of China's urbanization and the attainment of the overall goal of building a harmonious society. In recent years, governments at all levels have introduced various social security policies and initiatives for landless farmers. There are four typical models. The first is the Zhejiang model which mainly uses land for insurance and basic security by converting farmers into workers via employment training, establishing community shareholding economic cooperatives and leveling land replacement. The second is Shanghai "small town insurance model," the essence of which is "land for security." This model provides landless farmers with a lump sum basic old-age and medical insurance of no less than fifteen years, which, to a certain extent, addresses the needs of landless farmers for elderly care and major medical treatment in the protection of their basic interests. This model emphasizes "delivering the social security while helping them get employed" as the settlement policy, which changes farmers' traditional idea of security and encourages them to get employed in the market economy. The third is the Nanhai model of Guangdong, the core of which is to exchange farmers' land rights for the benefits of industrialization. The model extends farmers' long-term secure rights to their contracted land under the agricultural land contract system, which keeps the income and the added value of the land with the collectives and does not change the collective ownership of the land. It allows farmers to obtain the benefits of industrialization through the institutional innovation of "turning farmers into stockholders." The fourth is the Xianjia model of Hunan, the basic content of which can be summarized as "centralized resettlement and integrated development." The model transforms landless farmers into urban residents through comprehensive community management and guided transformation of community culture. Although these four typical models have their own advantages and disadvantages in terms of effectiveness, they provide

---

13 Ministry of Human Resources and Social Security and National Bureau of Statistics. "2007 Statistical Report on the Development of Labor and Social Security Programs." http://wl.mohrss.gov.cn/gb/zwxx/2008-06/05/content_240415.htm.

useful experience for solving the increasingly prominent problem of social security for landless farmers in China.

In addition to the above two special forms of social security, the Chinese government has also introduced, in recent years, policies to provide support to some rural households that practice family planning.

4 Urban-Rural Integration: the Goal of Rebuilding the Rural Social Security System

With the continuous improvement of China's socialist market economy, its powerful role in resource allocation has been brought into full play, featuring a large-scale cross-regional flow of labor mainly from rural to urban areas. Market-oriented reforms, industrialization and urbanization are promoting the integration of urban and rural areas and the creation of new combinations, which requires the connection of rural social security system with the urban one and eventually the establishment of a national social security system with the same standards for both rural and urban residents. However, as mentioned earlier, although China has created a basic framework of rural social security system, the characteristics of gradual reform and the path dependency of the traditional system have not fundamentally changed the overlapping of social security system with the production system in rural China. Explorations are still being made on the local level. Therefore, it is necessary to gradually develop a socialized rural social security system independent of the production system.

China is getting closer to the goal of building a rural social security system that is compatible with the socialist market economy after continuous reforms. Rural social security has changed from a temporary measure of poverty alleviation and relief to a new measure of "gradually forming a system that helps to promote social equity and justice." The goal is to change the rural social security system that overlaps with the production system and to "establish a social security system for both urban and rural residents" by 2020, as proposed by the Third Plenary Session of the 17th CPC Central Committee. Rural old-age insurance, new rural cooperative medical care, and minimum living allowances are fully promoted with related components of the social security system, which is gradually becoming standardized and institutionalized. The participation data show that the government, market entities and the private sector are all working together, and a diversified funding mechanism is taking shape. All the changes are evidence of the creation of a social security system outside of the rural production system, where standardized institutional arrangements replace the traditional family and land support in assuming responsibility for rural social security.

It should be noted that China's rural social security system is still far from being in place if measured by the goal of an integrated urban and rural social security system. China's rural social security system has a series of problems that need to be solved, such as limited coverage, low level of support, large gaps in funding sources, and overlapping management and functions. Therefore, the scope, structure, components and standards of the rural social security system should be set up according to the stage of economic development, the farmers' income difference and affordability. The reform should be continuously carried out by means of categorized design and step-by-step implementation.

The Third Plenary Session of the 17th CPC Central Committee has drawn a beautiful blueprint for the future of China's countryside – "extending the scope of public finance to cover rural areas and developing public programs for rural areas so that the majority of farmers have access to education, employment, medical care, elderly care and housing." The purpose is to ensure that farmers fully enjoy the fruits of China's reforms and development, and "to improve the rural social security system on the principle of broadening the coverage and ensuring the basic, multi-tiered and sustainable support."[14] Therefore, we have every reason to expect that, with the improvement of the rural social security system independent of the production system, a well-structured social security system covering both urban and rural areas will take shape in the near future.

14 "Decision of the Central Committee of the Communist Party of China on Several Major Issues Concerning Promoting Rural Reform and Development." http://cpc.people.com.cn/GB/64093/64094/8194418.htm.

CHAPTER 4

The Evolution of Disaster Relief Policies in the People's Republic of China

A Critical Analysis

*Jiang Jiwei**

Abstract

The disaster relief policies concern the direction and basic approach of disaster relief efforts. Since the founding of the People's Republic of China, the Chinese government has formulated different disaster relief policies at different times. The evolution of disaster relief policies shows a shift to more science-based operations and the new policies embody the modern disaster relief philosophy of involving both the government and the general public, defining responsibilities properly and putting people first. Overall, public participation in disaster relief operations, however, needs further exploration under the new policies.

Keywords

People's Republic of China – disaster relief policy – evolution

Every endeavor needs an overarching and strategic policy for its goal and direction. Disaster relief policies concern the direction and the basic approach of disaster relief efforts. Since the founding of the People's Republic of China (PRC), the Chinese government has formulated different disaster relief policies at different times. A close examination of these policies will be of positive significance to current and future disaster relief operations.

* Jiang Jiwei, J.D., associate professor at the Ministry of Education Training Base for College Counselors (South China Normal University).

 | DOI:10.1163/9789004737990_005

1 Establishing the Initial Disaster Relief Policies

1.1 *Natural Disasters in the Early Years of the PRC*

China is a vast country with complex geographical and climatic conditions, and natural disasters have occurred frequently since ancient times. "During the 3,703 years from 1766 BC to 1937, a total of 5,258 floods, droughts, locust plagues, hail, gales, earthquakes, frosts, snows and other disasters had occurred, averaging about one disaster every six months."[1] After the founding of the People's Republic of China in 1949, natural disasters continued to occur frequently. As Chen Qiyuan, then Vice Minister of Internal Affairs, summarized, "The disasters of 1949 were of many kinds (mainly floods), covering a wide area and lasting a long time. It was caused by not only the bandits of the United States and Chiang Kai-shek, but also the rule of the feudal class for a long time."[2] According to the statistics in *Cases of Major Natural Disasters 1949–2004*, seven of the fifty-three major natural disasters occurred from 1949 to 1956 during the fifty-five years after the founding of the PRC.[3] In addition, in the early years of the PRC, spring famine, drought, agricultural diseases and insect pests, hail, frost and other natural disasters struck frequently, causing huge losses and seriously hampering the country's economic and social development. In 1949 alone, floods affected an area of 127.87 million *mu* nationwide and about 45.55 million people in 498 counties and cities of 16 provinces and autonomous regions, causing the collapse of over 2.34 million houses and a reduction of 5.7 billion kilograms in grain production. In 1953, the area of affected crops nationwide reached 351.23 million *mu*.[4]

1.2 *The Self-Help Policy in the Early Years of the PRC*

In face of serious natural disasters, the CPC and the Chinese government immediately put disaster relief on the agenda and promptly formulated the

1 Deng Yunte. 1958. *A History of Disaster Relief in China*. Beijing: SDX Joint Publishing Company. 38.

2 "A Summary of Disaster Relief Efforts in the Past Year: A Report by Vice Minister of Internal Affairs Chen Qiyuan at the National Civil Affairs Conference on July 24, 1950." *The People's Daily*, September 13, 1950.

3 The seven major natural disasters that occurred between 1949 and 1956 were typhoon No.6 in 1949, floods in Jianghuai and North China in 1949, floods in the Huaihe River Basin in 1950, the Jianchuan earthquake in Yunnan in 1951, the flood in the Yangtze-Huaihe River Basin in 1954, the flood in 1956 and typhoon No.12 in 1956. Department of Disaster Relief, National Disaster Reduction Center, Ministry of Civil Affairs. *Cases of Major Natural Disasters 1949–2004*, August 2005. 1–47.

4 Department of Rural Welfare, Ministry of Internal Affairs. 1958. *Natural Disasters and Disaster Relief Efforts Since the Founding of the People's Republic of China*. Beijing: Law Press. 1.

disaster relief policy of "saving through disasters prevention, self-help through production, mutual assistance, and work-relief." In fact, this policy represented the CPC's consistent thinking and experience in dealing with natural disasters during the period of its regional governance. In 2012, the film *Back to 1942* drew the attention of the society to the problem of famine and gave us an idea of how differently the Guomindang (the Nationalists) and the CPC dealt with the problem. In 1942, a serious famine occurred in the Central Plains with Henan province as the center. In order to complete the task of purchasing grain, the GMD-led government blocked the information of disaster areas. In sharp contrast to the GMD government, the CPC launched a vigorous campaign of disaster and famine relief in the border areas, especially in the Shanxi-Hebei-Shandong-Henan border region, which suffered from the triple blows of drought and the attacks by Japanese soldiers and by the Guomindang army. The main approach was to combine government relief, mutual assistance and self-help to make the relief campaign an endeavor led by the border region government and involving all stakeholders in a mass campaign. Relief efforts were also combined with production activities of disaster victims. Various forms of mutual assistance and cooperation were introduced to help restore agricultural production to support rural sideline businesses and handicrafts. In fact, this model of disaster relief laid the foundation for early PRC's disaster relief policy.

The initial policy of "saving through disasters prevention, self-help through production, mutual assistance, and work-relief" was suitable in the early years when the PRC faced a shattered country with shortages of funds and supplies and money was needed on so many fronts. There was little money and material to aid the affected areas. Hence, the policy did not propose government relief funds and support for the affected areas, but prioritized disaster prevention. The inclusion of work-relief programs in the policy was made for the same reason of lacking relief funds but intended to involve the disaster victims in public works to ease the pressure of providing disaster relief funds.

On this basis, the first National Civil Affairs Conference in 1950 formally proposed the disaster relief policy of "self-help through production, frugal disaster management, mutual assistance, work relief, and relief provisions when necessary." Compared with the previous policy, this one emphasized the importance of self-help via production activities, and clarified the supporting role of the government in disaster relief. Therefore, it was a disaster relief policy featuring "self-help through production."

After the people's commune movement, people's communes, production brigades and production teams were set up in various places, making it possible to give full play to the strength of collective organizations in fighting against disasters. Therefore, the disaster relief policy was adjusted to "relying on the people and the collective power, focusing on self-help through production activities with the provision of necessary government relief." Although there were some differences in wording, this adjusted policy was similar to the previous one in that the focus was on self-help and the government relief was supplementary. On the whole, it was a more positive approach to disaster relief.

The reason that such a policy was adopted in the early years of the PRC was due to the limited economic and financial resources on one hand and the position of rural China in national industrialization strategy on the other hand. As noted in the *Directive of the Ministry of Internal Affairs on Strengthening Frugal Practice in Disaster Management in the Affected Areas*, "food production in the country at the time could not fully meet the needs of the government and the people, and the government could only devote a certain amount of resources to help the disaster victims in order to concentrate on the completion of national economic development plan."[5] Under the extremely difficult conditions at that time, the agricultural countryside was crucial to the implementation of the industrialization strategy. Self-help through production activities could reduce the financial burden on the government. More importantly, it helped maintain stability in rural areas, prevented the outflow of population, improved the productivity and purchasing power of rural residents, and provided raw materials, funding and the market for industrialization.

1.3 *Self-Help Initiatives and Effects in the Early Years of the PRC*

Under the guidance of the abovementioned policy, China adopted corresponding disaster relief measures.

1.3.1 Developing Sideline Businesses, i.e. Self-Help through Production

In this regard, the central government put forth the idea of making full use of local resources and encouraged mutual assistance, freedom of lending and loaning to address the shortage of funds. For the producers, the method was to loan the grains first and receive the finished products afterwards. For the transport service providers, the method was to loan the goods first and make the payment afterwards. Local trading companies and supply and marketing cooperatives entered into contracts with producers and sellers to promote local products. With sufficient funds and sales channels, rural sideline businesses developed very fast. In February 1951, about fifty percent of the households were engaged in sideline businesses in the hardest-hit areas of Hebei Province,

5 Policy Research Office of Ministry of Civil Affairs. *Compilation of Civil Affairs Documents* (II). September 1984. 88.

with better participation of sixty to seventy percent in some villages and even eighty to ninety percent in a few villages.[6] These sideline businesses increased the income of disaster victims and enhanced their self-help capacity.

1.3.2 Work-Relief Programs That Engaged Disaster Victims in Public Works

Compared to the simple cash payments and in-kind relief, this policy approached disaster management with practical and long-term benefits. In the early years of the PRC, the central government actively promoted work-relief programs, offering disaster victims various job opportunities on public works whenever feasible and possible. This measure proved fruitful in many places. The Chaobai River Lower Reaches project and the Golden Gate Canal project – the two largest water conservancy projects in Hebei Province that used this approach – "became the source of livelihood for 600,000 people for a whole month and was dubbed the 'life-saving project' by disaster victims."[7]

1.3.3 Frugal Practice and Mutual Assistance

A campaign "to save 50-gram rice" was launched among local government employees and the People's Liberation Army. Some government agencies even encouraged a daily reduction of 200 to 250 grams of rice per person with some officials donating all their allowances to the disaster victims. Regarding urban support for the disaster relief in the countryside, Xie Juezai noted that "only when the countryside overcomes the disaster and gradually reaches abundance can the cities recover more quickly" and "we hope that city people will continue to show their friendly support and respond enthusiastically to the disaster relief fundraising."[8] The shortage of relief supplies was promptly and effectively alleviated through disaster relief fundraising activities in major cities and the "one bowl of rice campaign" in villages.[9]

---

6 Department of Rural Welfare, Ministry of Internal Affairs. 1958. *Natural Disasters and Disaster Relief Efforts Since the Founding of the People's Republic of China*. Beijing: Law Press. 36.

7 "Report of the Party Leadership Group of the People's Government of Hebei Province on the Work of Spring Sowing and River Engineering to the Party Committee (June 1951)." Archives of Hebei Province: 907–15-4.

8 *Collected Works of Xie Juezai*. 1989. Beijing: People's Publishing House. 707.

9 The "50-gram Rice Campaign" and the "One Bowl of Rice Campaign" are two forms of disaster relief fundraising activities. The former was mainly conducted within government agencies and the People's Liberation Army, and the latter mainly in villages. "Report by Vice Premier Dong at the Inaugural Meeting of the Central Disaster Relief Committee." *The People's Daily*, March 7, 1950.

The disaster relief policies in the early years of the PRC played an important role in reversing the ineffectiveness of disaster relief efforts by historical dynasties. During the time of economic difficulties, the policy basically achieved the goal of "ensuring no one starves or freezes to death, no major epidemics break out, and no disaster victims leave the affected areas on a large scale." The basic needs of disaster victims were satisfied and production activities went on smoothly. In addition, water conservancy projects and the Huai River control project were effectively promoted amid the disaster relief efforts. Under the guidance of the disaster relief policies of this period, China made great achievements on the disaster relief front and gradually established a disaster relief and mitigation system led by the central government with many good practices that are still used today.

2 Re-adjustment of Disaster Relief Policies

2.1 *Complex Changes in Disaster Relief Policies*

From May 26 to June 18, 1958, the Fourth National Civil Affairs Conference was held under the auspices of the Ministry of Internal Affairs. The conference put forward the requirement that "disaster relief efforts must serve the Great Leap Forward in agricultural production and the eradication of natural disasters." It also established the disaster relief policy of "prioritizing prevention before relief, combining prevention and relief, relying on the collectives, making agriculture the mainstay while leveraging sideline businesses, and encouraging collaboration and frugal practice to eradicate disasters."[10] The biggest changes in this policy was twofold: one was to "combine prevention and relief" and "prioritize prevention before relief;" and the other was to eliminate natural disasters. Such changes occurred due to social and natural factors, first of all. Natural disasters had changed a lot in terms of frequency and scale compared to the early years of the PRC, so greater importance was put to disaster prevention. Secondly, the Ministry of Internal Affairs proposed that disaster relief should serve the agricultural leap forward, and disaster prevention could better fulfill this requirement in contrast to disaster relief. Lastly, the CPC and the Chinese government underestimated the impact of natural disasters due to such factors as the great achievements made in disaster relief in the early years of the PRC, the improvement of disaster prevention and relief capabilities after

10 "A Rising Wave of Social Welfare Production: The Fourth National Civil Affairs Conference Decides to Implement the General Line from Four Aspects." *The People's Daily*, June 30, 1958.

agricultural cooperative efforts, and the "Left" influence during the Great Leap Forward. A blind optimism changed the understanding of natural disasters in the early years and led to the wrong idea of eliminating natural disasters in a short period of time. For example, in the book *Historical Records on Natural Disasters and Disaster Relief since the Founding of the People's Republic of China* published at that time, it was pointed out that "famines are no longer a problem. In a few years, or a decade, people would not know what a famine is."[11] With such understanding, specialized disaster relief agencies were abolished, and some regions concealed or misreported disaster situations, which fostered a blind optimism from the central to local levels and led to a lack of precautions against serious natural disasters. This, coupled with the limited funds provided by the central government for disaster relief, weakened the capacity to respond to disasters and indirectly aggravated the severity of natural disasters. Some scholars, when studying the causes of the 1959–1961 famine, argue that the government's untimely relief efforts and poor relief ability were also the main factors leading to the famine and the varied intensity of the disaster across the country.[12]

Of course, although this policy caused late action in disaster relief, the proposed idea of "prioritizing prevention before relief" was more in line with the modern philosophy of disaster relief, and indeed produced some results in relief operations. Under the guidance of this policy, water conservancy and disaster prevention projects were carried out on a large scale, effectively preventing the occurrence of spring famines and droughts. The CPC and the Chinese government even organized discussions on the Three Gorges Project during which constructive ideas were put forward.

After the Cultural Revolution began, frequent political movements disrupted the organization of relief efforts, which were not given enough attention, and the Ministry of Internal Affairs, which was in charge of disaster relief, was abolished in October 1969. The disaster relief responsibilities initially assumed by the Rural Social Relief Department of the Ministry of Internal Affairs were assigned to the Central Agricultural Commission, the Ministry of Agriculture, the Ministry of Finance and other government agencies. The enormous changes in organizational structure had great impact on disaster relief operations, causing widespread disruption.

---

11 Department of Rural Welfare, Ministry of Internal Affairs. 1958. *Natural Disasters and Disaster Relief Efforts Since the Founding of the People's Republic of China*. Beijing: Law Press. 1.

12 Fan Ziying and Meng Lingjie. 2005. "A Review of Studies on the 1959–1961 Famine in China." *Jiangsu Social Sciences*, (2).

2.2 *Restoration and Adjustment of the Disaster Relief Policies*

In 1978, the Seventh National Civil Affairs Conference restored the disaster relief policy prior to the Cultural Revolution amid the reorganizational efforts and the beginning of reforms and opening up. On that basis, the Eighth National Civil Affairs Conference in 1983 changed the disaster relief policy to "relying on the people and the collectives, promoting self-help through production activities, encouraging mutual assistance, and seeking necessary relief and support from the government." Compared with previous disaster relief policies, the most significant feature of this new policy was the addition of "mutual assistance" and "government support." The introduction of this policy was inseparable from its historical background.

2.2.1 Notable Rural Changes

The implementation of the household contract responsibility system not only liberated the production forces, but also increased the enthusiasm of farmers for production. In addition, the industrial structure of the countryside changed. The contribution of sideline businesses to the total value of agricultural output increased every year, improving farmers' lives. With their income growing every year, their ability to help themselves was also enhanced, and they had the resources to provide relief. The disaster relief policy in the early years of the PRC also noted "mutual assistance," but it could only be simple cooperation in terms of labor and relief tools rather than material assistance, given the low living standards of farmers at the time.

2.2.2 Government's Introduction of Poverty Alleviation Policies after the Start of Economic Reforms

Disaster relief alone cannot lift the disaster victims out of poverty. It is imperative to combine "necessary relief" with "support." The support in policies, funds, technology, materials and other aspects for disaster victims will ensure that they continue to increase their income in the development of production and improve their ability to withstand and overcome disasters so as to fundamentally get out of poverty and be better off. Hence, the policy of government support and poverty alleviation was introduced to effectively combine poverty alleviation with disaster relief to enhance the effectiveness of disaster relief efforts.

2.2.3 Clarification of the Nature of Civil Affairs Work by the CPC and the Government

One of the highlights of the Eighth National Civil Affairs Conference was the definition of the nature of work on civil affairs. On April 9, 1983, Minister Cui

Naifu delivered a report entitled "Striving for a New Prospect in Civil Affairs under the Guiding Principles of the Twelfth CPC National Congress." It was pointed out in the report: "Civil affairs is about people. To carry out such work, we must not only have the support of the government, but also mobilize the people and rely on them." "The work on civil affairs is characterized by public participation, social engagement and diversity."[13] The clear definition of civil affairs work provided a theoretical basis for the socialized reform of disaster relief operations. In line with the idea of socialized reform, the disaster relief policy of 1983 still gave great importance to the practice of self-help through production and mutual assistance among people.

2.3 *Basic Measures of Government Support and Mutual Assistance*

2.3.1 Combining Disaster Relief and Poverty Alleviation

Historically, poverty and natural disasters have been inextricably linked. Poorer areas are usually weak in dealing with natural disasters but face more frequent occurrences of natural disasters. As a result, "a new disaster strikes before the victims recover from the impact of the previous one."[14] Conversely, the more disasters there are, the more devastating to society, and the poorer the victims become. Based on this understanding and in the context of rural poverty alleviation policy, the Ministry of Civil Affairs proposed that "poverty alleviation and disaster relief should be combined, and that disaster relief funds can be used to support poor households' production activities under the premise of ensuring the basic needs of disaster victims."[15]

2.3.2 Creating Rural Reserve Funds Associations for Disaster Relief and Poverty Alleviation

The reserve funds association is membership-based social security organization of mutual assistance at the basic level that pool together the money and grains from the farmers for the purpose of solving their own problems. In times of disasters, it would help affected members to solve their difficulties in terms of food, clothing, repairing houses and treating diseases. When there were no disasters, it can be used to support poor members in their efforts to develop production and address the urgent needs of other members. This actually

13 Policy Research Office of Ministry of Civil Affairs. *Compilation of Civil Affairs Documents* (I). September 1984. 30.

14 Li Wenhai. 2004. *History Is Not Far*. Beijing: China Renmin University Press. 209.

15 Policy Research Office of Ministry of Civil Affairs. 1986. *Selected Documents on Civil Affairs (1985)*. Beijing: Huaxia Publishing House. 104.

pushes the traditional practice of mutual help to a new level with a fixed form of organization, regular operations and established rules.

2.3.3 Changing the Usage of Disaster Relief Funds

"It is not only a delicate economic but also a political task to distribute disaster relief funds."[16] Since the founding of the PRC, the government had been adhering to the principle of free use of disaster relief funds. However, with the passage of time, this form of distribution revealed more and more drawbacks. It not only made disaster victims more dependent on the government, but also hindered the development of disaster prevention awareness among them. In addition, with the increase of rural personal income, disaster victims developed the ability to repay some or all of the relief funds. Therefore, the Ministry of Civil Affairs made some adjustment and combined paid use with free use of disaster relief funds. It not only expanded the relief coverage, but also aroused the enthusiasm of disaster victims for production activities and improved their disaster prevention awareness and self-help ability.

The adjustment of the disaster relief policy during this period led to some breakthroughs in China's disaster relief efforts. It not only ensured meeting the basic needs of the victims, but also improved the efficient use of relief funds. More importantly, China gained rich experience in the reform of disaster relief operations, raised the self-help awareness of the victims, and aroused the enthusiasm of local governments for disaster relief. Of course, the adjustment of disaster relief policy was closely related to the country's economic strength and financial system. The policy adjustment in this period featured the stress on mutual assistance and government support. Apparently, with the deepening of reforms and opening up, the country's economic strength had been enhanced, which was reflected in the corresponding growth in government support for disaster relief. However, as the reform was still in the stage of "crossing the river by feeling the stones," the country's economic strength was still not yet very great. Therefore, the government had to reduce the pressure by improving the efficient use of limited disaster relief funds, such as the contractual use of funds, the combination of paid and free use of funds, and the trial application of disaster relief insurance.

16 Policy Research Office of Ministry of Civil Affairs. September 1984. *Compilation of Civil Affairs Documents* (II).. 103.

3 Reform of Disaster Relief Policy

The change in disaster relief policy in 1983 was considered as an adjustment here because the change was rather small compared with the policy established in the early PRC. The focus had remained on self-help through production activities, but the thinking of government relief policy shifted from passive relief to active support. The policy changes thereafter were considered as reforms here because those changes were indeed all-round and profound.

3.1 *Establishing a New Disaster Relief Policy*

The disaster relief policy of 1983 remained unchanged over a long period of time. It was not until the 12th National Civil Affairs Conference, held in 2006, that a new formulation was made. In his speech at the conference, Vice Premier Hui Liangyu proposed a disaster relief policy featuring "government leadership, tiered management, mutual assistance and self-help through production activities" and noted the need to improve the emergency rescue system and the quality of disaster relief operations.[17] The policy was once again explained by Minister of Civil Affairs Li Xueju in 2007. He said: "Due to global warming and frequent occurrence of extreme weather events, disaster mitigation and relief efforts are faced with serious challenges. We should fully enforce the *Law on Emergency Response*, implement the policy of 'government leadership, tiered management, mutual assistance and self-help through production activities,' focus on increasing the capacity for emergency response and comprehensive disaster mitigation, improve the disaster response mechanism, build disaster response capacity and raise the level of disaster mitigation and relief."[18] This policy seemed simple, but its implications were far-reaching, as it echoed the philosophy of modern disaster relief.

In fact, the turning point between the old and new policy came at the 10th National Civil Affairs Conference held in 1994, although this policy was proposed in 2006. Prior to 1994, because of the government's limited financial

17 Hui Liangyu. "Studying and Implementing the Guiding Principles of the Sixth Plenary Session of the Sixteenth CPC Central Committee and Giving Full Play to the Fundamental Role of Civil Affairs in Building a Harmonious Society – Speech at the 12th National Civil Affairs Conference." Website of Ministry of Civil Affairs of the People's Republic of China. http://www.mca.gov.cn/article/zwgk/mzyw/200711/20071100003827.shtml. October 15, 2013.

18 Li Xueju. "Comprehensively Implementing the Guiding Principles of the 17th CPC National Congress and Pushing the Development of Civil Affairs to New Stage from a New Historical Starting Point." China Social Welfare Network, http://shfl.mca.gov.cn/article/ldjh/200809/20080900019844.shtml. October 15, 2013.

resources, the only way to alleviate the financial pressure was to improve the efficient use of disaster relief funds when there was not a large increase in the amount of disaster relief funds. Such an approach was clearly transitional in nature. The so-called "support" was mainly provided for the old revolutionary base areas, areas with large ethnic minority populations, and border and poor areas; but due to the limited resources in those areas, the support funds may not necessarily have achieved the desired results. It was naturally difficult to recover the funds; hence, the financial pressure on the central government remained enormous. In addition, as the financial management system with "multi-tiered contract responsibility" became increasingly incompatible with the socialist market economy, the central government decided to reform the financial system and start adopting a tax-sharing system on January 1, 1994. This move allowed local finance to grow rapidly. The 10th National Civil Affairs Conference was held in such a context, further recognizing the idea of involving the public in disaster relief. Minister of Civil Affairs Duoji Cairang noted: "The work on civil affairs involves many tasks which cannot be accomplished by the government alone, so the general public must be involved. It should be changed from government initiative to the people's action." The conference also advocated the establishment of a tiered management system for disaster relief operations. Premier Li Peng said in a discussion with the conference participants: "How can we address the basic needs of the affected population? I think the main responsibility lies with the provincial governments, and a provincial system should be established, with subsidies from the central government." "Provincial governments should play a leading role, establishing relief funds and allocating funds for places where natural disasters are more frequent."[19] In view of the above two points, the 10th National Civil Affairs Conference was actually a prelude to the later reform of the disaster relief policy. After more than ten years of exploration, a new disaster relief policy was finally established at the 12th National Civil Affairs Conference in 2006, ushering in a new stage of science-based regular disaster relief operations.

3.2 *Implications of the New Disaster Relief Policy*

First, highlighting the responsibility of a modern government.

What exactly is the government's position and responsibility in disaster relief? In the previous disaster relief policies, the focus was on self-help through production activities, with the government playing only a supporting role. In reality, however, the government was in charge of everything, and

19 Legal Affairs Office of Ministry of Civil Affairs. 1995. *Selected Documents on Civil Affairs (1994)*. Beijing: China Social Publishing House. 19, 5, 6.

its responsibilities were not clearly defined. The 15th CPC National Congress offered a clear guideline on the institutional reform of the State Council, namely "separating government administration from enterprise management and streamlining agencies." The principles for the institutional reform were also clarified, namely "transforming government functions and separating government administration from enterprise management according to the requirements of socialist market economy, adjusting organizational structure of the government in the principle of streamlining and efficiency, adjusting the responsibilities and powers of government departments, clearly dividing responsibilities among departments, and improving the administration mechanism, and strengthening the administrative system in the principle of law-based government administration."[20] Taking this opportunity, the Ministry of Civil Affairs decided to implement an institutional reform to transform its functions and raise the level of public participation in disaster relief. The Ministry of Civil Affairs asked local civil affairs departments to "transform their functions, gradually extricate themselves from the routine work, and focus their efforts on macro-management, issuance of policies, formulation of laws and regulations and standardization of services to fully mobilize the enthusiasm of various social organizations, mass organizations and volunteers in providing disaster relief services and to entrust them with certain routine work and gradually promote public participation in disaster relief operations.[21]

In the process of involving the public in disaster relief, the government has made clear its role and responsibility as the guiding leader. It means that the government will free itself from the specific affairs of disaster relief and play its role in the following two aspects. One is to provide financial support. Over the past 30 years of reform and opening up, China's economic strength has increased unprecedentedly, and it has become the second largest economy in the world. Compared with the pre-reform period, the government has the ability to increase the financial investment in disaster relief and play a leading role in this regard. The other is to regulate and coordinate disaster relief efforts. In other words, the government should play the role of a commander, coordinator and supervisor in disaster relief. To involve the public in disaster relief does not mean to reduce the government's responsibility for disaster relief. From the perspective of public administration, disaster relief is an important part of

---

20 Literature Research Office of the CPC Central Committee. 2000. *Selected Important Documents since the 15th CPC National Congress* (Volume 1). Beijing: People's Publishing House. 242.

21 Legal Affairs Office of Ministry of Civil Affairs. 1999. *Selected Documents on Civil Affairs (1998)*. Beijing: China Social Publishing House. 371–372.

public affairs, and government leadership is a reflection of not only the government's basic functions but also its protection of basic human rights. From an economic perspective, this is also consistent with the government's role in providing public goods. In fact, the Chinese government's leadership over disaster relief efforts fits well with the country's current system and characteristics, and can effectively enhance the efficiency, especially the speed of disaster relief.

Second, clarifying the responsibilities of central and local governments for disaster relief.

When we say that the government takes charge of everything in disaster relief, it mainly refers to the central government. In other words, there is no clear division of responsibilities between central and local governments. Local governments, close to disaster relief sites, have failed to take up their due responsibilities. Financial input from the central government has always been the dominant relief in major, medium and minor disasters, as well as in emergency relief during disasters, post-disaster recovery, reconstruction and living arrangements for the victims (see Table 4.1).

After the National Conference of Civil Affairs Department (Bureau) Directors in 1996, local governments at all levels accelerated the pace of implementing the tiered management. In 1996, thirty provinces, municipalities and autonomous regions listed the "217 item" in their budget;[22] and the coverage was a hundred percent at the municipal level in twenty-one provinces and more than ninety percent at the county level in fourteen provinces, and up to a hundred percent at the county level in eight provinces. A total of 2,203 counties

TABLE 4.1 Central and local government spending on disaster relief, 1981–1995 (unit in 0.1 billion)

Time period	National disaster relief funds	Central government relief funds	Local relief funds
"6th Five Plan"	35.2	27.1	8.1
"7th Five Plan"	56.4	51.3	5.1
"8th Five Plan"	94.1	82.9	11.2

SOURCE: *CHINA STATISTICAL YEARBOOK ON CIVIL AFFAIRS (2006)*. CHINA STATISTICAL PUBLISHING HOUSE, 2006, PP. 85–86.

22 "217" is a unified code for funds used by central and local governments for spending on natural disasters.

listed the "217 item," accounting for 76.4 percent of all counties in the country.[23] Local governments not only budgeted for disaster relief, but also invested more resources each year. In 2000, for example, the central government spent over RMB 3.18 billion on disaster relief while local governments allocated over RMB 1.57 billion, an increase of 45.7 percent over 1999, in addition to measures to promote self-help and mutual assistance. All this consolidated the material foundation of government-led disaster relief.[24] Tiered assignment of responsibilities at the local level is a modern idea of disaster relief, which is more reasonable and orderly in terms of division of labor.

Third, adding new contents to self-help through production activities

Self-help through production activities was a basic principle of disaster relief established in the early years of the PRC. It was an important measure to alleviate the financial difficulties and material shortages at the time. Today, although the material and physical conditions have greatly improved, the principle of self-help through production should be continued. Disaster victims are best familiar with the disaster sites and know the fastest access to the sites, which is a special advantage for minimizing the casualties. Self-help through production not only shows the public nature of civil affairs but also help to reduce the victims' dependence on the government. It is of great importance in mobilizing the disaster victims to engage in the work of post-disaster recovery and reconstruction. Disaster victims are not just the recipients of aid, but are also the participants in disaster relief activities. The government and other sectors' attention and help are all external factors, but post-disaster recovery and reconstruction eventually depend on the victims themselves. Therefore, the mindset of the victims is particularly important in disaster relief. Self-help through production activities fosters exactly this positive mindset in disaster relief. The importance of self-help through production activities is, therefore, examined not just from the material perspective, but more importantly from the perspective of people's mindset in post-disaster recovery and reconstruction.

Fourth, making disaster relief an endeavor of the public

Previous disaster relief policies stressed mutual assistance among the people, but the CPC and the Chinese government did not fully understand the role of the government and the nature of philanthropy with the biased view that developing charity and encouraging mutual assistance discredited

23 Legal Affairs Office of Ministry of Civil Affairs. 1998. *Selected Documents on Civil Affairs (1997)*. Beijing: China Social Publishing House. 305.

24 Legal Affairs Office of Ministry of Civil Affairs. 2002. *Selected Documents on Civil Affairs (2001)*. Beijing: China Democracy and Legal System Publishing House. 313–314.

socialism. Therefore, the government took care of everything in disaster relief. This phenomenon was gradually improved after the beginning of reforms and opening-up, especially in the 1990s, when public participation in disaster relief efforts began to be recognized by the whole society. In his visit to Shaanxi and Gansu provinces at the end of 1995, President Jiang Zemin said that people should collect clothes, quilts and articles of daily use in the cities to support and help the people in poverty-stricken areas, making it a regular activity of voluntarism in the society. To that end, the Ministry of Civil Affairs and the State Council's Leadership Group for Poverty Alleviation and Development jointly issued the *Opinions on Organizing Regular Donations in Large and Medium Cities to Support Disaster-affected and Poverty-stricken Areas*, requiring "the start of a 'Support the Poor' campaign in 1996 with the donation of clothes and quilts in large and medium-sized cities across the country."[25] Donations by the public have since become regular and organized, effectively making up for the insufficiency of the government in disaster relief.

Under the guidance of the new disaster relief policy, China has made great achievements in both material and non-material support in disaster mitigation and relief efforts. On the material front, the central and local governments have increased their disaster relief funds, whereby the amount of public donations has shown a trend of steady growth, and the reserve of relief supplies has been gradually replenished. On the non-material front, disaster mitigation and relief operations have become more scientifically implemented with established rules. According to statistics, since 1978, two hundred million people have been relocated, along with their wealth in tens of billions of yuan over the thirty years. In short, with the country's growing economic strength, the Chinese government has greatly increased its capacity for disaster mitigation and relief, especially for emergency relief. China's successful disaster relief efforts have won worldwide acclaim.

An examination of disaster relief policies adopted since the founding of the PRC shows that China's disaster relief policy has been improving, and the new policies feature modern ideas of disaster relief, such as effective interactions between the government and the people, proper division of responsibilities, and the focus on people. While recognizing China's achievements, we should also be clear-headed that further explorations need to be made in promoting public participation in disaster relief in China. To date, such participation has been mainly in the form of making donations. More diversified approaches should be introduced. For example, public participation in disaster relief

25 Legal Affairs Office of Ministry of Civil Affairs. 1997. *Selected Documents on Civil Affairs (1996)*. Beijing: China Social Publishing House. 313.

should be comprehensively promoted in such realms as raising disaster relief funds, distribution of funds, reserves of supplies, donation receiving institutions, disaster relief entities, and disaster relief information. Only in this way can the power of the private sector be released to the greatest extent in a disaster relief system marked by interactions between the government and the people.

CHAPTER 5

Is Food Security an Issue for China or for the World?

The International Perspective

Zhu Huaxiong and Qu Shang *

Abstract

International researches on China's food security have been shifting along with the changes in the world since the founding of the People's Republic of China. The perspectives of international scholars on China's food security have transitioned since the 1990s from primarily China's domestic food security to the relations of China's food security with global food security, as China is increasingly integrated with the global economy with its rapid economic growth and steady population rise. The study of China's food security is now placed in the framework of global food security, making China's food security an important part of global food security.

Keywords

food security – international research – shift

China's food security has always been an important issue of interest to foreign scholars, given the fact it is a big country with a huge population. Since the founding of the People's Republic of China (PRC), the focus of foreign scholars' research on China's food security has changed along with the country's development, but the scope of their research has been basically limited to China's domestic food security. Since the economic reforms and opening-up, China has been gradually integrated into the global economic system, and its food security has become an integral part of global food security. This paper attempts to sort out the results of overseas research on China's food security.

* Zhu Huaxiong, Ph.D. in economics and associate professor at Zhongnan University of Economics and Law; Qu Shang, Ph.D. in economics and professor at Zhongnan University of Economics and Law.

 | DOI:10.1163/9789004737990_006

1 Initial Attention to China's Food Security

In 1949, when the Guomindang government in Nanjing was defeated and retreated to Taiwan, the U.S. government published a white paper titled "United States Relations with China", which attributed Guomindang's failure in the mainland partly to the country's large population and its failure in feeding the population. Therefore, according to the white paper, the failure of the U.S.-supported Guomindang government was not due to the United States nor the Guomindang government to some extent, but due to the overpopulation of China, "an issue that no government has managed to solve so far."[1] This was the starting point of overseas research on China's food security.

Mao Zedong refuted the aforementioned view of the U.S. government. He pointed out clearly that the root cause of the failure of the Guomindang government in the mainland was its corruption and reactionary rule. The U.S. government had expected that the Communist Party of China (CPC) would not be able to solve the economic problems on its own but to rely on American flour and become an American colony as the solution to China's food problem. On behalf of the CPC, Mao Zedong promised: "A new China will emerge soon with a large population, abundant natural resources, high living standards and an advanced culture."[2] Mao's words provided an important inspiration for the country's endeavor to promote economic recovery and development with a focus on grain production to ensure food security in the PRC.

2 Studies on China's Planned Grain Procurement and Marketing Policy and on the Quota Policy of Production, Procurement and Marketing

Foreign scholars started the studies of the motivation behind China's introduction of the planned grain procurement and marketing policy relatively early and have achieved more research results in this regard. They approached the issue mainly from economics and paid more attention to the connections between economic phenomena.

Dwight Perkins examined the necessity of planning the procurement of grain and other consumer goods from such perspectives as lacking investments

1 Party Literature Research Office of the CPC Central Committee, ed. 1991. *Selected Works of Mao Zedong* (Volume 4). Beijing: People's Publishing House. 1510.

2 Party Literature Research Office of the CPC Central Committee, ed. 1991. *Selected Works of Mao Zedong* (Volume 4). Beijing: People's Publishing House. 1510–1512.

in agriculture, ideology and political control. He was among the first foreign scholars who noted the pressure on grain market due to the strategy of prioritizing heavy industry.[3] The same view can be found in the book *Cambridge History of China: The People's Republic (1949–1965)* edited by John K. Fairbank and Roderick MacFarquhar. According to the book, top priority was given to industrialization under the strategy of developing heavy industry first to catch up with other countries. Therefore, when food crisis occurred in the autumn of 1953, the government adopted the policy of planned grain procurement at fixed prices and increased the pace of developing agricultural production cooperatives, instead of using the price adjustment mechanism, due to concerns about the growth of government revenue, the increase or decrease of investments in the means of production, and the supply of consumer goods to farmers.[4]

Kenneth Walker reviewed the development of the planned grain procurement and marketing policy during the 1953–1962 period and the late 1970s. He estimated the quantity of grain procured and marketed within provinces, between provinces and between urban and rural areas, and attempted to assess the policy's impact on grain consumption.[5] According to Li Fuzhong, a Chinese scholar from Taiwan, the "top CPC leaders (probably Mao Zedong himself) were already thinking about introducing the planned grain procurement and marketing policy even before the food crisis in 1953." He further put forward the view that the purpose of the policy was to ensure grain export.[6]

Thomas Bernstein carried out a study on the background and purpose of the introduction of quota-based grain production, procurement and marketing policy in 1955. He focused on the critical role played by the primary-level officials in China's political system and the difficulties they faced in bridging the high-level authorities and the general public. He examined the causes of the food crisis in the spring of 1955 and analyzed the mechanism of mass campaigns in rural China.[7] According to Huang Zongzhi's empirical research,

3 Dwight H. Perkins. 1968. *Market Control and Planning in Communist China*. Cambridge and Massachusetts: Harvard University Press. 42, 205–214.

4 J. K. Fairbank and R. MacFarquhar, eds. 1991. *Cambridge History of China: The People's Republic (1949–1965)* (trans: Wang Jianlang). Shanghai: Shanghai People's Publishing House. 169–185.

5 Kenneth. R. Walker, 1984. *Food Grain Procurement and Consumption in China*. Cambridge: Cambridge University Press.

6 Li Fuzhong. 2003. "Why did the Communist Party of China abandon New Democracy?" *Journal of the Institute of Modern History, Academia Sinica* 40: 198–217.

7 Thomas P. Bernstein. 1970. "Cadre and Peasant Behavior under Conditions of Insecurity and Deprivation: The Grain Supply Crisis of the Spring of 1955," in A. Doak Barnett, ed. *Chinese Communist Politics in Action*. Seattle and London: University of Washington Press. 365–399.

in the countryside of the Yangtze River Delta region, "the quota-based grain production, procurement and marketing policy not only incorporated small-scale farming into national planning, but also led farmers to the road of collectivization."[8] T. J. Hughes and D. E. T. Luard argued that farmers' grain reserves and the flood of 1954 caused serious food shortages in 1955, and the quota-based grain production, procurement and marketing policy was to consolidate the planned grain procurement system, rather than to make the system more flexible or to relax the government's quota requirements, for the Chinese government did not procure too much grain in 1954.[9] Vivienne Shue did not agree with the view. She compared the changes in the quantity of government-procured grain before and after the introduction of the quota-based grain production, procurement and marketing policy, and held that the policy reflected the country's reduced demand for grain, instead of the government's attempt to become more stringent.[10]

3 Causes of China's Three-Year Economic Hardship

China suffered severe economic hardship and a great famine during the three years from 1959 to 1961. Foreign scholars have long shown interest in the famine, but they did not conduct systematic research until the 1980s due to limited information available. They achieved some impressive research results in the 1990s, bringing foreign research of China's food security to the first climax.

The earliest research result was the paper, "Stalinism, Famine, and Chinese Peasants: Grain Procurements during the Great Leap Forward," published in 1984 by Thomas Bernstein of Columbia University. According to the paper, grain procurements increased significantly because of false reports of grain output. The proportion of government-procured grain rose sharply from 25 percent to 39.7 percent in 1959 and 35.6 percent in 1960 while grain output in 1959 actually dropped by more than thirty percent compared with 1958. Therefore, the cause of the Great Famine was the government's overemphasis

8 Philip C. C. Huang. 2000. *The Peasant Family and Rural Development in the Yangzi Delta, 1350–1988* (trans: Cheng Hong, Li Rongchang, and Lu Hanchao). Beijing: Zhonghua Book Company. 175.

9 T. J. Hughes and D. E. T. Luard. 1959. *The Economic Development of Communist China, 1949~1958*. London: Oxford University Press for the Royal Institute of International Affairs.

10 Vivienne Shue. 1980. *Peasant China in Transition: The Dynamics of Development Toward Socialism, 1949~1956*. Berkeley: University of California Press. 236.

on grain procurement.[11] In the 1990s, Penny Kane conducted a comprehensive study of the causes and the scope of the Great Famine and its impact on Chinese population and society, drawing the attention of international community to China's food security, government policies and economic development strategy.[12] According to Nicholas R. Lardy, belief in the grandiose reports of grain output during the Great Leap Forward led to a 13 percent reduction in the planned farming in 1959. This resulted in a corresponding reduction of 13 percent, or about twenty-five million tons, in grain output. Such wrong decision-making was an important cause of the serious food shortage at the time.[13]

According to Justin Yifu Lin and others, as members of the people's communes did not have the right to withdraw from the commune and it was impossible to prevent laziness, some members could easily slack off and impair the efficiency in the use of resources. The institutional defect of the people's commune system was the root cause of the Great Famine.[14] Zhang Xin and Wen Guanzhong established a model based on empirical inference, which included all factors related to the Great Famine. They held that none of the factors concerning production were directly related to the occurrence of the Great Famine which was caused not by the decrease in grain supply or the government's grain allocation, but by the irrational consumption behavior of public canteens.[15] Yang Dali's further research questioned why the Great Famine in 1959 was not effectively contained and became even worse in 1960? He argued that the deep-seated cause of the Great Famine was political, while other factors such as public canteens and people's communes were only part of a series of extreme policies during the Great Leap Forward and they did not count as the only causes of the Great Famine.[16]

---

11 Thomas P. Bernstein. 1984. "Stalinism, Famine, and Chinese Peasants: Grain Procurements during the Great Leap Forward." *Theory and Society* 3: 339–377.

12 Penny Kane. 1993. *Famine in China 1959–1961: Demographic and Social Implications* (trans: Zheng, Wenxin et al.). Beijing: China Social Sciences Press.

13 J. K. Fairbank and R. MacFarquhar, eds. 1991. *Cambridge History of China: The People's Republic (1949–1965)* (trans: Wang, J. L.). Shanghai: Shanghai People's Publishing House. 402–404.

14 Justin Yifu Lin. 1984. "Collectivization and China's Agricultural Crisis in 1959–1961." *The Journal of Political Economy* 6.

15 Chang Gene Hsin and Guangzhong James Wen. 1997. "Communal Dining and the Chinese Famine of 1958~1961." *Economic Development and Cultural Change* 1.

16 Dali L Yang. 1996. *Calamity and Reform in China: State, Rural Society, and Institutional Change Since the Great Leap Famine.* Stanford, Calif.: Stanford University Press.

Other studies on China's food security conducted by foreign scholars during this period included "Chen Yun's Strategy for China's Development: A Non-Maoist Alternative" by Nicholas R. Lardy and Kenneth Lieberthal,[17] "Agriculture in China's Modern Economic Development" by Nicholas R. Lardy,[18] and "Studies on the Population of China, 1368–1953" by Ping-ti Ho.[19] These studies addressed a wide range of issues, including economic development strategy during the Great Leap Forward, the quantitative relationship between grain procurement and consumption, economic policies that neglected agricultural development, government's inaction on disaster relief with the ongoing Great Leap Forward, and events such as the Lushan Conference.

It should be noted that there are two deficiencies in the studies conducted by foreign scholars. One is that they did no empirical study of China's climate from 1959 to 1961. Their analysis of political and ideological factors lacks the support of important factors of natural conditions. The other is that they use Western theories and paradigms to analyze the specific events in China, which has the issue of applicability to China's realities.

4 What Makes China's Food Security a Global Issue?

At the beginning of reform and opening up, China attached great importance to grain production and its grain output increased substantially. With the shift of economic reform from the focus on the rural to the urban areas, however, agricultural production and grain output were stagnant between 1985 and 1989. China's food security issue had not been solved once and for all. Foreign studies on China's food security during this period were mainly conducted from the perspective of China's grain import and the research scope was limited to China itself as its grain import had little impact on grain prices at international markets at the time.

As China opened up wider to the outside world and its economic strength grew, Chinese economy became increasingly integrated into the global economy. Foreign scholars' attention was once again drawn to China's food security and the issue began to be examined in a global context. In 1993, Australian

17 Nicholas R. Lardy and Kenneth Lieberthal, eds. 1983. *Chen Yun's Strategy for China's Development: A Non-Maoist Alternative.* Armonk, New York: M. E. Sharpe, Inc.

18 Nicholas R. Lardy. 1983. *Agriculture in China's Modern Economic Development.* Cambridge: Cambridge University Press.

19 Ping-ti Ho. 1989. *Studies on the Population of China, 1368–1953* (trans: Ge Jianxiong). Shanghai: Shanghai Ancient Books Publishing House.

scholars Ross Garnaut and Ma Guonan used the income elasticity coefficient to revise the data for grain rations and GDP per capita in the base period, and projected China's grain supply and demand based on the historical data for food consumption structure changes in some Asian countries and regions with the same consumption preferences.[20]

From August to September 1994, Lester Brown, President of the Worldwatch Institute, published three influential articles on China's food security in *The Washington Post*, *World Watch* and *International Herald Tribune*, bringing foreign research on China's food security to the second climax. Brown then went on to promote his views at several important international conferences and kept adding new evidence. Based on the experiences of Japan, South Korea and Taiwan of China, Brown put forward the view implying that as China continued to industrialize and arable land decreased with water resources increasingly scarce and income levels rising, China's food shortage would skyrocket to about two hundred million tons, which was the volume of global food trade at the time. He predicted that China's food shortage would reach 374 million tons in 2030. He even argued that "in the integrated global economic system, a rise in China's food prices would lead to a surge in world food prices, China's lack of arable land would become a problem for the world, and China's water shortage would also affect the world." The Chinese would scramble for food from the rice bowl of the world; China would become a major burden to the world; and China's food crisis would evolve into the world's food crisis.[21]

This was the first time that foreign researchers put China's food security in the analytical framework of global food security, associating China's food security with its international responsibility. The shift suggests that China's food security has become an integral part of global food security in the new historical context of economic globalization and the research on China's food security has taken on international significance. It also shows that China can no longer be excluded from global affairs in the process of economic globalization. Moreover, Brown's equating China's food security to global food security proposes a "China threat" theory, which has been strongly refuted by scholars around the world including Chinese scholars and the Chinese government.[22]

---

20 Ross Garnaut and Ma Guonan. 1993. *Grain in China: A Report*. Beijing: China Agricultural University Press.

21 The three articles are "How China Could Starve the World: Its Boom Is Consuming Global Food Supplies", "China's Future Grain Shortage", and "Question for 2030: Who Will Be Able to Feed China?".

22 Liang Ying, ed. 1996. *Can China Feed Itself?* Beijing: Economic Science Press; State Council Information Office of China. 1996. "White Paper on China's Grain Problem." *The People's Daily*, October 25; Ke, B. S. 1995. *China's Grain Market and Policy*. Beijing: China Agriculture

After Brown, the "China threat" theory had a new addition of "China's food security threat".

In the late 1990s, with the decrease of agricultural land, China had more shortage of food production resources. In the meantime, high-speed economic development worldwide brought about the increase of people's income and consumption levels and the upgrade of consumption structure, pushing up global food prices. Developed countries of Europe and the United States, in order to reduce the pressure of rising oil prices on the costs of domestic products, successively promoted bio-energy programs and reduced grain exports from 2005, increasing the shortage of the global grain supplies. Two global food crises have occurred since the beginning of the 21st century.

On May 2, 2004, *The New York Times* published an article entitled "China Races to Reverse Its Falling Production of Grain." According to the article, although many economists saw the government's focus on food production as inopportune and uneconomical in an era of economic globalization, China's rapid urbanization was devouring the land of millions of farmers and millions more of farmers had given up growing food because it was not profitable. The situation made Chinese leaders worry about the country's ability to feed itself, prompting an urgent move to rein in the loss of land so as to increase food production. This policy highlighted the importance of food security for China. Moreover, China's 1.3 billion people needed to be fed by seven percent of the world's arable land.[23] To solve China's food security is to solve the problem of feeding twenty-two percent of the world's population. Therefore, China's food security is far from being a matter for the Chinese themselves. It concerns the future of China and the world. China will make a great contribution to global food security by solving its own food security problems.

At the critical juncture of the global food crisis in 2007–2008, some developed countries once again pointed the finger of blame at developing countries such as China and India, with China in particular. They argued that the Chinese were consuming more beef and beef production consumed more grain, thus causing a global food shortage. According to a research report published by Biofuels Digest on May 1, 2008, China's annual per capita meat consumption was fifty-three kilograms, 1.12 times that in 1995. That would require an increase of nearly two hundred million tons of feed grains and eventually lead to the depletion of the world's food stocks by 2010. The shutdown of all ethanol plants in the United States would delay the depletion until 2013. The report

Press; Chen, Y. B. 1995. *Studies on China's Grain Development*. Beijing: All-China Federation of Industry and Commerce Press.

23 Hu Yuemin. 2006. *On the Future Food Security of China*. Beijing: Science Press.

also noted that China's per capita meat consumption was forty-five percent less than that of the United States, and if Chinese people ate as much meat as Americans, the world would need an additional 277 million tons of feed grain and sixty-eight million acres of arable land. Therefore, the surge in global food prices was caused by China's massive grain imports, and the global food crisis was caused by Chinese people's starting to eat meat.[24] This argument completely ignores the fact that developed Western countries consume far more meat than developing countries. It regards the rising living standards of the Chinese people and the people of other developing countries as the source of the global food crisis, so as to shirk their responsibility for running bioenergy programs that caused the global food crisis.

Investment bank Merrill Lynch's monthly economic report on China refuted the theory of "China's food security threat." The report argued that the impact of meat on the grain trade was mainly linked to the trade in animal feed such as corn and soybeans. In terms of the trade in corn, China's corn export was only twelve percent of that of the United States from 2001 to 2007. Although China's corn export reached its peak in 2002, it was still less than the average annual increase in corn consumed by ethanol production in the United States between 2001 and 2007, during which the proportion of corn produced for ethanol production in the country rose from less than eight percent to nearly twenty percent of its total corn production. China's share in the international trade of corn was not big, so its impact on global corn prices was rather limited. In fact, the increase or decrease in feed consumption has little effect on corn prices compared with corn consumed by biofuels. Since the beginning of the 21st century, industrial corn consumption in the United States has been soaring year by year and its growth reached 24.69 million tons during 2007–2008, which was 1.6 times the total corn feed consumption in Southeast Asia (15.4 million tons) and 51.33 percent of the total feed consumption in the twenty-seven EU countries (48.19 million tons). It is fair to say that the increase or decrease of feed consumption has a negligible impact on corn prices. By contrast, corn prices have soared in recent years largely because of the rising demand for corn for ethanol production in the United States. Therefore, the energy policy of the developed world, not China, is the culprit in this round of rise in global food prices.[25]

---

24 The United States claims that changes in the consumption structure of emerging markets such as India and China are the main cause of rising global food prices. "Global Food Crisis", http://www.jrjg.com/redian/lswj/lshwj.html.

25 Ma Junqin. "Chinese People's Eating More Meat Causes the World's Food Shortage? The Merrill Lynch Report Refutes It." *National Business Daily*. http://www.jrjg.com/neirong/look.asp?id=xinwen_08050816350_69506.

Some foreign researchers hold the opinion that with the rapid growth of China's economy comes a huge demand for energy. In the process of converting grain into bioenergy, China has appropriately liberalized the import of oil products such as soybeans on the basis of increasing self-sufficiency in main grains such as rice, wheat and corn to ensure the food security of itself and the world. Other researchers argue that China has stepped up its energy diplomacy by promising African countries to curb rising food prices in order to secure supplies of energy such as crude oil in Africa. If China buys a large amount of grain on international markets, it will surely drive up global grain prices and directly impact African countries. Therefore, China will remain basically self-sufficient in grain production, instead of buying large quantities of food from international markets.[26]

In light of rapid economic growth, the Chinese government has intensified efforts to develop alternative energy sources, tightened controls on grain-based ethanol production, restricted the use of edible grains such as corn as raw materials for biofuels, and encouraged the biofuel industry to "focus on non-grain products." Apparently, the government has placed food security in a more important position. Since 2003, China has implemented a new agricultural policy, abolishing agricultural taxes, raising grain purchase prices, banning the indiscriminate seizure of farmland, and increasing agricultural investment to offset the rising prices of seeds, diesel oil, fertilizers and pesticides. China's grain output has increased steadily. It has once again stressed that at least ninety-five percent of its agricultural products should be produced domestically and that food security is a priority for the country.[27]

Since the mid-1990s, the research on China's food security has become one of the focuses of attention in the world, and China's food security has become an integral part of global food security. Therefore, Chinese researchers on food security should engage more in exchanges with their international counterparts on China's food security research to clear up misunderstandings, refute fallacies and work with them in addressing the issue of food security.

---

26 "Will China Become a Corn Importer?" *Reference News*, May 13, 2010.

27 "An Outline of National Plan for Medium – and Long-Term Food Security (2008–2020)", November 13, 2008. http://www.gov.cn/jrzg/2008-11/13/content_1148414.htm.

CHAPTER 6

The Emergency Response Mechanism in the Early Days of the People's Republic of China

A Case Study of the Plague Control in Chabei Prefecture in 1949

*Li Honghe**

Abstract

The outbreak of plague across Chabei Prefecture of Chahar Province in October 1949 was a major health emergency immediately after the founding of the People's Republic of China (PRC). The Chinese government acted quickly with investigation and assessment of the overall situation and set up the mechanism of political mobilization, decision-making and information exchange. These measures provided good experience for policymakers and practitioners to manage similar health emergencies later in the country and laid the solid foundation for the development of China's healthcare and social progress.

Keywords

early days of the People's Republic of China – Chabei Prefecture – plague – emergency response mechanism

An emergency is a serious situation or event that occurs unexpectedly that threatens or will potentially threaten people's life and property and the social order and stability. The suddenness, uncertainty and great damage involved make the emergency response and the response mechanisms extremely important. The outbreak of plague across Chabei Prefecture of Chahar Province in October 1949 was a major emergency, which tested the governing capability of the CPC and the government.

* Li Honghe, associate professor at School of Politics and Management Science, Henan Normal University.

 | DOI:10.1163/9789004737990_007

1 The Outbreak and Spread of the Plague in Chabei Prefecture

Plague is a severe infectious disease caused by the bacterium Yersinia pestis. It has a high mortality rate and can wreak havoc on society. Existing studies show that it occurred frequently in North China in modern times, with the outbreaks in 1917, 1929, 1931 and 1942 the deadliest. Shortly after the founding of the PRC, a plague epidemic broke out in Chabei Prefecture, causing heavy death tolls. The plague passed through the following stages:

1.1 *Latency*

The plague in Chabei Prefecture originally started in mid-July 1949. The first incidence was reported in Qianyinkou village where three villagers died. Because local herdsmen lacked the knowledge of hygiene and did not attach sufficient importance to the outbreak, it spread to Chahan Bengbeng village in Kangbao District of Chabei Prefecture.[1] At the beginning of October 1949, the bubonic plague transformed into the pneumonic plague, and people infected with pneumonic plague could die in one day or 3–5 days. With the spread of the plague, the number of deaths gradually increased. Sometimes, six deaths were reported in one day. By October 19, Chahan Bengbeng village had reported 36 deaths.[2]

1.2 *Acceleration*

After the plague outbreak in Chahan Bengbeng village, villagers panicked and fled the village, bringing the disease to other places. Around October 20, 1949, Shenwan Qingyingzi reported six deaths, Beisha Chengzi reported seven deaths, Lizhandi village reported three deaths, and Nanjinggou reported one death.[3] Cases were also reported in Baoyuan and Duolun. The plague soon spread throughout Baoyuan county and then struck Zhangbei and other places. On October 25, it spread from Zhangbei to the vicinity of Zhangyuan. In early November, it spread to Jining in Suiyuan Province. Just over half a month after it was found in Qianyinkou village of Chahar League, the disease spread to Chahan Bengbeng village, Kangbao, and Jijiafang village in the southeast of

1 Lü Guangming. Due to timely control and lockdown, the plague in Chabei Prefecture has been brought under control and Zhangjiakou City will launch a large-scale rat control campaign after vaccination. *The People's Daily*, November 13, 1949.

2 A letter from a farmer in Chahan Bengbeng Village, Inner Mongolia, to thank the Soviet medical workers for helping to fight the plague, *The People's Daily*, November 7, 1951.

3 Lü Guangming. Due to timely control and lockdown, the plague in Chabei Prefecture has been brought under control and Zhangjiakou City will launch a large-scale rat control campaign after vaccination. *The People's Daily*, November 13, 1949.

Zhangjiakou. It spread to 10 villages within more than 150 kilometers from the place where it first started. With 69 people infected and 66 deaths reported, the plague posed a great threat to life.[4]

1.3 *Eradication*

After November 5, 1949, no more victims of the plague were found in the affected areas. On November 11, the Central Government Council held the fifth administrative meeting. Dong Biwu made a report, confirming that the plague in the affected area had been brought under control in the past week.[5] On November 15, the Central Disease Prevention and Control Committee, on the basis of in-depth studies, submitted an action plan to the Central People's Government for approval, requesting to open the Datong-Nankou section of the Beijing-Baotou Railway from November 16 and "remove part of the cordon sanitaire in Chanan." Since then, the transportation of materials between Chahar, Suiyuan and various places became smooth. "Due to the fact that the plague in Chabei Prefecture, Chahar League and Jijiafang village in Zhangjiakou has been brought under control," it was decided that schools, movie theaters, open-air markets and other businesses and venues in Zhangjiakou City would reopen on November 16.[6] After December, the plague in Chabei Prefecture was completely eradicated, the lockdown was lifted, signaling the end of the prefecture's fight against the plague.

2 Plague Response Mechanism and Its Operation

The outbreak of plague in Chabei Prefecture in October 1949 put the CPC and the Chinese government to a serious test. The biggest challenge was to build a comprehensive emergency response mechanism that would integrate

4 Guang Ming: The Central Disease Prevention and Control Commission submitted a petition to the Government Council. Jingsui Road has been reopened. The Chabei cordon sanitaire has been partially removed. Strict quarantines will be kept in place because the plague has not ended. *The People's Daily*, November 16, 1949.

5 The Government Council held its fifth government meeting and decided to build the East China Working Group to provide guidance for the takeover of the Wang Jingwei regime. Vice Premier Dong reported that the spread of the plague had been stopped. *The People's Daily*, November 12, 1949.

6 Guang Ming: The Central Disease Prevention and Control Commission submitted a petition to the Government Council. Jingsui Road has been reopened. The Chabei cordon sanitaire has been partially removed. Strict quarantines will be kept in place because the plague has not ended. *The People's Daily*, November 16, 1949.

research, decision-making, publicity, education and public engagement, with the goal to minimize the damage and improve the efficiency and effectiveness of emergency response.

2.1 *Political Mobilization Mechanism*

Political mobilization is a movement in which the ruling party or government utilizes its political resources to organize people to work for economic, political, and social development goals.[7] The successful control of the 1949 plague in Chabei Prefecture resulted from the political mobilization by the Chinese government, which involved two factors: the government's efforts to mobilize citizens, and the citizens' response to government's call to participate in sanitation and rat eradication campaigns.

Epidemic prevention is a matter of public interest. The government must mobilize people to participate and play an active role of creativity and initiative-taking. On October 25, 1949, Zhang Su, chairman of the government of Chahar Province, held a cadre meeting in Zhangbei County to convey the provincial party committee's resolution. Zhang Su first explained the seriousness of the plague, calling on members of the party, the government and the military as well as the civilians to "take immediate action to eradicate the plague" and emphasized that in order to eradicate the plague, both the affected and non-affected areas should launch campaigns to eradicate plague vectors–rats and fleas.[8] A few days later, the North China Bureau of the Central Committee of the CPC issued a notice, pointing out that the plague was a deadly disease that was spreading very rapidly. The railways connecting Beijing, Tianjin, and Zhangjiakou that the military and civilians frequently traveled on was very likely to spread the disease to Hebei, Beijing and Tianjin. Therefore, government agencies in Beijing and Tianjin should make effective preparations on the ideological, organizational, and medical fronts to protect the capital from the plague.[9] On October 29, the People's Government of North China and the North China Military Region jointly issued an order requiring that "the military and civilians in the affected area immediately prioritize plague eradication." The people's governments of all provinces and municipalities and

7 Lin Shangli. 2000. *A Study of Political Forms in Contemporary China.* Tianjin People's Publishing House. 271.

8 Lu Guangming. Chairman Zhang Su of Chahar Province personally visited Chabei Prefecture to engage the whole of society in the fight against the plague. After returning to Zhangjiakou, he talked to our reporter about the plague in Chabei. *The People's Daily*, October 30, 1949.

9 The North China Bureau issued a notice on the urgency of plague control. The plague in Chabei is spreading Zhangjiakou. Relevant authorities of Beijing and Tianjin should make effective preparations. *The People's Daily*, October 28, 1949.

the provincial military regions should urge subordinate units to participate in plague prevention.[10] On October 30, *The People's Daily* published an editorial, stating that "the outbreak of plague in Chabei and Inner Mongolia have attracted wide attention. The fight against the plague has begun, and eradicating the plague should become the current top priority for the people of North China."[11]

People in North China took immediate actions in response to the government's call to fight the plague. In addition to holding a military meeting, setting up a plague prevention committee, and drawing up a plague prevention plan, the Beijing Army General Hospital organized an internal sanitation and vaccination campaign. Students of the Medical School of Peking University discussed the government's call and agreed that fighting plague was not only their responsibility but also the touchstone of their commitment to "serving the people wholeheartedly." The faculty association of departments and hospitals put out posters to enthusiastically answer the government's call and was ready to dispatch staff members to fight against the plague at the frontline.[12] On October 28, the Central Disease Prevention and Control Committee designated the Tiantan Disease Prevention and Control Center as the producer of plague vaccines, and the staff of the center unanimously promised that they would do their best to complete the task. They said: "There are no armed enemies in North China, but the plague is just as vicious as armed enemies. We must resolutely and thoroughly eradicate it north of the Great Wall!" All the employees of the center were in high spirits, with branches of trade unions and production units holding meetings, studying production plans, setting up production targets for groups and individuals, and committing workers to production targets with organized competitions at work.[13] In order to completely eradicate the plague, Zhangjiakou, Beijing and other places launched large-scale rodent control campaigns. The rodent control campaign in Zhangjiakou City was carried out under the guidance of the Soviet animal expert Kamenev. The rodent control team consisted of 122 students from North China Medical

10 "The North China People's Government and the North China Military Region jointly issued a plague control order." 1949. Xinhua Bookstore Editorial Department (ed.), *Starting the Fight Against Plague*. 6.

11 "Starting the Fight Against Plague." *The People's Daily*, October 30, 1949.

12 Peking University Medical School Communication Group. "Army General Hospital and Other Medical Facilities Are Ready to Fight the Plague at Any Time." *The People's Daily*, November 2, 1949.

13 Liu Junxiang. "The Disease Prevention and Control Office of the Temple of Heaven Plans to Expand the Production of Vaccines and Strives to Eradicate the Plague North of the Great Wall." *The People's Daily*, October 30, 1949.

University, Zhangjiakou Middle School, and other schools, who were divided into 10 groups. On November 9 and 10, they visited every household to inspect and block mouse holes and raise people's awareness about the importance of killing rodents and fleas. Data showed that the rodent control team inspected 2,897 houses in two days and found 4,033 rat holes. Rat capture began on November 12. Affected villages used home-made flea traps (sticky paper with a mixture of soybean oil, sesame oil, and rosin on it) to catch fleas, which proved very effective.[14] The Beijing Municipal Disease Prevention and Control Committee launched a rodent control campaign to prevent plague. The first phase of the campaign started in mid-November and ended on November 24. A total of 42,231 rats were caught in the city within 14 days. In the campaign, residents not only actively provided assistance to the authorities but also showed their creativity and inventiveness. For example, a local resident named Zhang Shanrui invented the "Wooden Cat", which caught more than 20 rodents in three days.[15] In early December, Beijing started the second phase of the rodent control campaign and achieved remarkable results.

2.2 *Decision-Making Mechanism*

The decision-making mechanism is at the core of an emergency response system. Decision makers need to respond immediately after the occurrence of an emergency, find a solution promptly and make decisions decisively to stop the deterioration of the situation. After the plague outbreak in Chabei Prefecture in October 1949, the decision-making mechanism was established for emergency response in the following way:

2.2.1 Establishing a Decision-Making Body for Plague Control

After the plague occurred in the Chabei Prefecture, the prefectural CPC committee responded quickly. On October 21, it called upon all party members, soldiers, and cadres to take upon themselves the responsibility of saving lives and mobilizing citizens in the fight against the plague in a calm and tenacious manner. The prefecture promptly established the plague control headquarters, with plague control organizations set up at the county, district, and village levels to oversee plague control efforts.[16] On October 24, the party,

---

14 Lü Guangming. "Due to Timely Control and Lockdown, the Plague in Chabei Prefecture Has Been Brought Under Control and Zhangjiakou City Will Launch a Large-Scale Rat Control Campaign After Vaccination." *The People's Daily*, November 13, 1949.

15 "The First Phase of the Rat Eradication Campaign in Beijing Has Ended." *The People's Daily*, December 1, 1949.

16 "Chabei Issued a Lockdown Order and Built a Plague Prevention Headquarters to Engage the Citizens in the Fight against the Plague." *The People's Daily*, October 28, 1949.

government, and military departments of Chahar Province met urgently to discuss plague control measures. At the meeting, it was unanimously agreed that the plague was the most vicious enemy of the people in the province, and that plague control was their current top priority. The Plague and Eradication Committee of Chahar Province was established, and it was decided that Chabei Prefecture and its counties should set up command centers to coordinate plague control efforts.[17] On the same day, the Chabei Prefectural CPC Committee held a cadre meeting. Officials of directly affiliated agencies and relevant departments and agencies of the government of Zhangbei county participated in the meeting. They emphasized the severity of the plague and mobilized public officials to participate in the fight against the plague. The cavalry divisions, the county brigades and militias of the Chahar Military Region set up roadblocks in designated areas.[18]

The CPC Central Committee showed great concerns for the plague. On October 27, the Central People's Government Council held a plague control meeting and rolled out a series of emergency response measures. In addition to the adoption of emergency response measures, the Council established the Central Disease Prevention and Control Committee, which was composed of Dong Biwu, Nie Rongzhen, Teng Daiyuan, Lu Dingyi, Li Dequan, He Cheng, and Yang Qiqing, and headed by Dong Biwu. After the plague control meeting was over, the committee immediately held its first meeting and decided to establish an office, a blockade division, a plague prevention division, a publicity division, and a secretariat with standard operating procedures.[19] On October 28, the Central Disease Prevention and Control Committee held a meeting and decided to launch a large-scale publicity campaign by immediately sending a brigade to the affected areas to support local plague control efforts.[20] Many CPC organizations, government departments and agencies,

---

17 Plague Epidemic Hit Chabei. The northern part of Chahar Province activated the emergency response mechanism. Chairman Zhang Su personally visited the affected area and dispatched the northeast plague prevention and control team to Chabei. *The People's Daily*, October 27, 1949.

18 Plague Epidemic Hit Chabei. The northern part of Chahar Province activated the emergency response mechanism. Chairman Zhang Su personally visited the affected area and dispatched the northeast plague prevention and control team to Chabei. *The People's Daily*, October 27, 1949.

19 To fight the plague in Chabei and prevent its spread, the Government Council held an emergency meeting and decided to impose strict traffic restrictions and send personnel to the affected area to support local plague response. The Central Disease Prevention and Control Committee with Dong Biwu as the top leader. *The People's Daily*, October 28, 1949.

20 The Central Disease Prevention and Control Committee convenes a meeting to mobilize people to fight the plague in Chabei and determine the list of personnel and their

and people's organizations in Beijing and other cities also participated in the fight against the plague. The Beijing Municipal People's Government held an interim meeting on October 28 to discuss plague control measures. Zhang Youyu reported on the outbreak and spread of the plague in Chabei Prefecture and the countermeasures adopted by the government. The Beijing Municipal People's Government decided to establish the Beijing Municipal Disease Prevention and Control Committee, with Mayor Nie Rongzhen as the director, with people from all walks of life invited as members of the committee or its standing committee to oversee the plague prevention and control in Beijing.[21] The establishment of plague control organizations at all levels of the government (from central to local) was of decisive importance for the successful eradication of plague in Chabei Prefecture.

2.2.2 Building Plague Control Teams to Support and Provide Guidance for the Affected Areas

After receiving the plague report from Chabei Prefecture on October 26, the Central Government Council met immediately and decided to send a brigade to the affected areas to support local plague control efforts. The plague control brigade, consisting of 727 medical workers from the Health Department of the Central Military Commission, the Northeast China Disease Prevention and Control Team, the Disease Prevention and Control Team of Inner Mongolia, the North China Disease Prevention and Control Team, the North China Medical School, the North China People's Hospital and other institutions, was immediately dispatched to the affected areas. The Central Plague Control Brigade was divided into three teams. After arriving in Zhangyuan, the first and second teams went deep into the affected areas. The third team mainly worked in Zhangyuan City and Jijiafang village located in the Jinjiang suburban area of the city. Some members of the third team worked in Jining and Datong.[22] The North China Disease Prevention and Control Department of the Central Military Commission and the Health Department of the Chahar Military Region jointly built a 20-person plague control team and went to Zhangbei

responsibilities, and sends three plague response teams to the affected areas. *The People's Daily*, October 29, 1949.

21 To prevent plague from spreading to the capital, Beijing establishes a plague control committee, and imposes quarantine in Xizhi, Chaoyang, and Yongding. *The People's Daily*, October 29, 1949.

22 Lin Hong. With strong government leadership and support of Soviet experts, the plague in Chabei has drawn to an end and the country has successfully prevented the plague from spreading to the capital, and the focus of plague control work has shifted to universal and permanent eradication of plague. *The People's Daily*, November 28, 1949.

with radio communications equipment and vaccines. They set off from the affected area on October 27 and inspected north-south transportation routes between Kangbao County and Zhangbei City, with Zhangbei City as their center of activities.[23] The 37-person plague control team built by the Health Department of the Inner Mongolia Autonomous Government was divided into a laboratory group, a rat capture group, a disinfection group, and a treatment group. On October 29, they went to the area where the plague started in Chabei Prefecture for in-depth investigations.[24] The central and local disease prevention and control teams actively launched publicity and education activities on the plague and other infectious diseases in the affected areas and achieved remarkable results.

2.2.3 Launching a Vaccination Campaign and Adopting Scientific Plague Control Measures

In the early days of the People's Republic of China, the mortality rate of the plague was very high. At a time when a quick cure was difficult to get, vaccination was a good way of prevention. On October 26, 1949, 77 members of the Northeast and North China Disease Prevention and Control Teams arrived in Zhangjiakou City, carrying vaccines for 50,000 people, to help Chahar Province fight the plague.[25] On October 31, 150 members of the second team of the Central Plague Control Brigade arrived in Zhangjiakou City, carrying plague vaccines and penicillin manufactured by the Soviet Union for more than 230,000 people. They participated in vaccination, disinfection, and rodent and flea control activities in Chahar Province and Inner Mongolia.[26] Since November 7, twenty-three vaccination teams composed of 136 medical workers from the Central Plague Control Brigade and Zhangjiakou City had been providing vaccination services in the urban area of Zhangjiakou. Data showed

---

23 Lü Guangming. Chairman Zhang Su of Chahar Province personally visited Chabei Prefecture to engage the whole of society in the fight against the plague. After returning to Zhangjiakou, he talked to our reporter about the plague in Chabei. *The People's Daily*, October 30, 1949.

24 The Central Disease Prevention and Control Committee calls on relevant departments to launch a plague prevention and control awareness campaign. The plague response team of Inner Mongolia inspected the source area of the outbreaks. *The People's Daily*, November 2, 1949.

25 The North China Bureau issued a notice on the urgency of plague control. The plague in Chabei is spreading Zhangjiakou. Relevant authorities of Beijing and Tianjin should make effective preparations. *The People's Daily*, October 28, 1949.

26 Lü Guangming. The plague response team arrived in Chahar. Zhangjiakou City started a universal vaccination program. The pneumonic plague has spread to the rural areas of Zhangjiakou City. *The People's Daily*, November 1, 1949.

that, on the evening of November 8, more than 93,800 people were vaccinated.[27] As of November 10, thanks to the hard work of the central and local disease prevention and control teams, more than 130,000 people of the city's more than 160,000 population, apart from those who were physically unfit for vaccination, were vaccinated against plague, drawing the vaccination campaign to a satisfactory end.[28] The vaccination campaign was crucial for raising the immunization rate in the affected areas and curbing the recurrence and spread of the plague.

2.2.4 Locking Down the Affected Areas and Imposing Traffic Restrictions across the Country

Following the plague outbreak in Chabei Prefecture, the CPC, government, and the military units of Chahar Province held an emergency meeting on October 24, 1949 and issued a series of traffic restrictions. They decided to draw two cordons from Duolun to Huade (along the border of Inner Mongolia and Chabei Prefecture) and along the Great Wall. People were not allowed to enter or exit the area between the two cordons, unless they went through a physical examination to obtain a special pass. Transportation (including vehicles and cattle) between Zhangjiakou and Chabei was immediately stopped. "The affected areas, villages, and households were quarantined, and people in surrounding villages were vaccinated." "People in the cordoned off areas were mobilized to ensure everyone would comply with the travel restrictions, not to come into contact with outsiders, or allow outsiders to stay overnight in the cordoned off areas."[29] The Health Department of the Municipal Government of Beijing immediately adopted emergency response measures after being informed of the plague outbreak in Chabei Prefecture and near Zhangjiakou. Starting from October 27, all long-distance buses and passengers from Zhangbei had to pass the inspection at Yongdingmen, Chaoyangmen, or Xizhimen before entering Beijing city. Inspection stations were set up at these three gates to inspect

---

27 Lü Guangming. More than one hundred medical workers in Zhangjiakou City participated in the fight against plague. Nearly one hundred thousand people received plague vaccine shots. School teachers are on a mission to debunk superstitions. *The People's Daily*, November 11, 1949.

28 Lü Guangming. Due to timely control and lockdown, the plague in Chabei Prefecture has been brought under control and Zhangjiakou City will launch a large-scale rat control campaign after vaccination. *The People's Daily*, November 13, 1949.

29 Plague Epidemic Hit Chabei. The northern part of Chahar Province activated the emergency response mechanism. Chairman Zhang Su personally visited the affected area and dispatched the northeast plague prevention and control team to Chabei. *The People's Daily*, October 27, 1949.

vehicles and passengers days and nights. Individuals with suspected or confirmed plague would be immediately placed under medical isolation at hospitals specializing in infectious disease.[30] In order to prevent the spread of the plague, the Beijing-Tianjin Railway Bureau decided to suspend service of Train No. 421/422 traveling between Beijing and Baotou, Train No. 423/424 between Beijing and Zhangjiakou, Train No. 425/426 between Beijing and Suizhou from October 27.[31] After the plague spread to Jining, the Central Disease Prevention and Control Committee immediately responded to the emergency and blocked the traffic between Datong and Fengzhen.[32] At the same time, three cordons were set up in Chabei Prefecture to temporarily stop people from entering or exiting the cordoned off areas, thus stopping the spread of the plague to other regions.[33] Promptly cordoning off affected areas and imposing traffic restrictions were the key to curbing the rapid spread of acute infectious diseases such as the plague.

2.3 *Information Exchange Mechanism*

In addition to establishing the basic information transmission elements in an emergency such as the bottom-up reporting and the top-down chain of command, the Chinese government, in the process of plague control in Chabei Prefecture, also launched a large-scale health and plague prevention publicity campaign to debunk superstitions and requested support and assistance from the Soviet Union and international organizations. Following the plague outbreak, the Chabei Prefectural CPC Committee immediately sent medical workers to the affected villages to publicize plague prevention and control knowledge. They organized, inspected, and oversaw local plague control operations. On November 1, the Central Disease Prevention and Control Committee issued the *Instructions on Public Communications of Plague Prevention and Control*, requiring local publicity departments and disease prevention and control departments to work closely together. They were expected to make good use of newspapers, radio stations, movies, publications, and other media forms to raise public awareness and engagement. The main task

30 To prevent plague from spreading to the capital, Beijing establishes a plague control committee, and imposes quarantine in Xizhi, Chaoyang, and Yongding. *The People's Daily*, October 29, 1949.

31 Six Beijing-Zhangjiakou and Beijing-Baotou trains are suspended to prevent the spread of the plague. *The People's Daily*, October 28, 1949.

32 The plague spreads to Jining. The Central Disease Prevention and Control Committee makes an emergency action plan and issues an order to block traffic between Datong and Fengzhen. *The People's Daily*, November 1, 1949.

33 *The Biography of Dong Biwu (1886–1975)*. 2006. Central Party Literature Press. 686.

of public communication was to disseminate the characteristics and dangers of the plague, the effects of plague prevention and its importance and necessity, the knowledge and methods plague prevention, and sharing experience in plague eradication, updating the epidemic status and prevention to make people of all walks of life realize the danger of the plague with high alert and all measures of prevention and control.[34] The Publicity Department of the Central Disease Prevention and Control Committee ran an education program on plague prevention and control, which was aired at Xinhua Broadcasting Station from 19:00 to 19:30 every day between October 31 and November 5. Broadcasting stations of Zhangjiakou, Chengde, Guisui, Taiyuan, Tianjin, Baoding, Tangshan, and other cities also participated in a simulcast.[35] In response to the call of the Central Government Council and the North China Bureau of the CPC to fight the plague, the North China Film Management Company screened the educational short film "How to Prevent Plague," produced by the Northeast China Film Studio, in every cinema in Beijing starting from October 29, to increase citizens' knowledge of plague prevention.[36] On November 2, *The People's Daily* published an article that reported the fight against the plague in Northeast China from several aspects such as rodent capture and control, flea control, vaccination, quarantine, disinfection, blockade, isolation and treatment as experiences to benefit other people in plague prevention.[37]

Mao Zedong was very concerned about the plague in Chabei Prefecture. On October 28, he notified Stalin and the Soviet government of the serious plague, requesting the assistance of Soviet medical workers.[38] Stalin agreed. Four Soviet medical experts, including Dr. Luo Guojin (as he is known in China), and a 32-person Soviet plague prevention team arrived in Beijing on the night of November 4 and the morning of November 5. They arrived in Zhangjiakou City on the evening of November 5 to support local plague control efforts. Dr. Luo Guojin and the team leader Maiysky conducted field investigations in Chahan Bengbeng village, Longwang Temple, and other affected areas. Plague expert

34 The Central Disease Prevention and Control Committee calls on relevant departments to launch a plague prevention and control awareness campaign. The plague response team of Inner Mongolia inspected the source area of the outbreaks. *The People's Daily*, November 2, 1949.

35 Beijing Xinhua Radio Station broadcasts messages about plague prevention and control. *The People's Daily*, October 31, 1949.

36 Cinemas in Beijing are playing plague related films. *The People's Daily*, October 29, 1949.

37 Introduction of North China's Plague Prevention and Control Experiences. *The People's Daily*, November 2, 1949.

38 *Manuscripts by Mao Zedong after the Founding of the People's Republic* (Volume 1). 1987. Central Party Literature Press. 98.

Dr. Lakson said during a program broadcast by Zhangjiakou People's Radio that "The plague in the PRC is about to be terminated." Maiysky introduced how to prevent plague on the radio. They played a certain role in popularizing scientific prevention and stopping the spread of the plague.[39]

3 Assessment of the Chabei Prefecture's Plague Response Mechanisms

The plague that occurred in Chabei Prefecture in October 1949, shortly after the founding of the RPC, did not cause tens of thousands of casualties like previous plagues. As the first plague that the PRC faced, however, it tested the leadership and governance of the CPC and the government. When the plague occurred, the CPC and the government calmly responded in the following ways.

First of all, they investigated to find out how things really stood. The relevant party, government, and military units of Chahar Province met on October 21, 24, and 25 discussed how to respond to and control the plague. The CPC Central Committee and the Central Government Council communicated with the governments of the affected areas and held meetings on October 27 and 28. They listened to the reports from the Ministry of Health and the health departments of Chabei Prefecture, analyzed the pattern of plague development, and quickly grasped the fundamental information of the plague.[40]

Secondly, they scientifically assessed the situation and carried out scientific demonstrations. After listening to the opinions of health, transportation, publicity, and other departments, the CPC Central Committee, the Central Government Council, and the party and government officials of Chahar Province carefully analyzed the nature and possible consequences of the plague outbreak, and quickly established the Disease Prevention and Control Committee, which included as members Vice Premier Dong Biwu, Mayor of Beijing Nie Rongzhen, Minister of Railways Teng Daiyuan, Minister of the Central Publicity Department Lu Dingyi, Minister of Health Li Dequan, Vice Minister of Health He Cheng, and Vice Minister of Public Security Yang Qiqing, to oversee the control of the plague. The establishment of the committee laid a solid foundation for effective decision making.

Third, they demonstrated political wisdom and took decisive actions. The plague occurred suddenly and might have caused a lot more of damage

39 Li Zhizhong. Soviet experts and plague prevention teams went to Inner Mongolia support local plague control. *The People's Daily*, December 20, 1949.

40 *The Biography of Dong Biwu (1886–1975)*. 2006. Central Party Literature Press. 686–687.

if the government had failed to act promptly and made informed decisions. Measures taken included sealing off the traffic to prevent the plague from spreading, sending medical workers and drugs to the affected areas, instructing the Ministry of Health to produce publicity materials and mobilize local newspapers, radio stations, movie theaters, and publicity teams to disseminate relevant knowledge and information, establishing plague prevention and control institutions with regular offices, and engaging the public in sanitation campaigns and campaigns to control rodents and fleas.[41] These actions were taken to safeguard public interests, protect lives, maintain social stability, and promote development. They pointed out the clear direction on how to win the fight against the plague.

Chinese government and the people also drew lessons from the plague in Chabei Prefecture and its successful eradication for subsequent emergence responses. Effective practices adopted by Chabei Prefecture in the plague fight in October 1949, such as launching health and disease prevention publicity campaigns, rolling out prevention-oriented policies, promoting vaccination, improving immunization rate, blocking traffic and implementing isolation rules, were widely promoted by the Ministry of Health and local health and disease prevention departments. In February 1950, the Ministry of Health and the Health Department of the Military Commission demanded that southeastern provinces where the plague was likely to occur in the spring "isolate patients on the spot and lock down the affected villages."[42] On November 25, 1950, Beijing promulgated the *Interim Measures for the Prevention of Infectious Diseases*, which stipulated that "patients with plague, cholera, smallpox, and encephalitis lethargica should be put in isolation at hospitals specialized in handling infectious diseases or other public and private hospitals designated by the public health authority."[43] Chabei Prefecture's handling of the affected areas during the 1949 plague offered an effective model for plague control afterwards. In 1955, Inner Mongolia basically followed the plague fight procedures of Chabei Prefecture in the 45 plague-affected areas, and quickly put the

41 To fight the plague in Chabei and prevent its spread, the Government Council held an emergency meeting and decided to impose strict traffic restriction and send personnel to the affected area to support local plague response. The Central Disease Prevention and Control Committee with Dong Biwu as the top leader. *The People's Daily*, October 28, 1949.

42 Instructions of the Ministry of Health of the Central People's Government and the Department of Health of the Military Commission on Military and Civilian Disease Control and Prevention during the Spring. *Voice of Doctors in Northern Anhui*. 1950 (2).

43 "Beijing Interim Measures for the Prevention and Treatment of Infectious Diseases." *Beijing Municipal Affairs News*, 1951 (8).

plague to an end.[44] It is worth noting that since the founding of the PRC to the present, the CPC and the Chinese government have calmly dealt with all kinds of issues and emergencies not only in health and disease prevention but also in the political, economic and diplomatic fields, due to the good use of the experiences accumulated in the early days of the PRC. During the SARS epidemic in 2003, the CPC and the Chinese government decisively adopted mobilization and comprehensive prevention measures to curb the spread of the epidemic. The measures they took during the SARS epidemic had many similarities to those of the plague prevention measures taken by Chabei Prefecture in the early days of the PRC.

The spread of plague in Chabei Prefecture also exposed low public awareness about public health and safety at the time. The plague occurred as early as mid-July 1949, but local herders, who lacked general hygiene knowledge, did not report it. Ignorance and superstition were prevalent problems at the time. After the death of many villagers in Chabei Prefecture, local people were afraid of burning the corpses. They did not report the deaths, or buried the dead secretly, which increased the difficulty of fighting the plague.[45] In some affected areas, people believed the plague had been brought by the Plague God. They tried to expel the plague through superstitious practices such as chanting prayers, burning incenses, and carrying out rituals of exorcism.[46] In response to the above-mentioned challenges, the CPC Central Committee, the Government Council and Chahar Province, Beijing and other local governments sent health publicity personnel to visit local residents, and expand their knowledge of plague prevention, which significantly facilitated the battle against the plague.

In summary, the 1949 plague in Chabei Prefecture was an emergency that occurred shortly after the founding of the PRC. The CPC and the government were effective in handling the emergency. The emergency response mechanism proved effective and reasonable. The successful experience in fighting the plague laid a solid foundation for the development of public health and social progress in China.

---

44 Liu Jiyou et al. 1997. *A Brief History of Plague Epidemics in Inner Mongolia*. Inner Mongolia People's Publishing House. 266–267.

45 Lü Guangming. Chairman Zhang Su of Chahar Province personally visited Chabei Prefecture to engage the whole of society in the fight against the plague. After returning to Zhangjiakou, he talked to our reporter about the plague in Chabei. *The People's Daily*, October 30, 1949.

46 Lü Guangming. More than one hundred medical workers in Zhangjiakou City participated in the fight against plague. Nearly one hundred thousand people received plague vaccine shots. School teachers are on a mission to debunk superstitions. *The People's Daily*, November 11, 1949.

CHAPTER 7

The Campaign against Opium and Other Drugs in Hebei Province in the Early Years of the People's Republic of China

*Dong Xiangqian**

Abstract

Before the founding of the People's Republic of China, exploitative foreign capital and incompetent domestic regimes gave rise to the cultivation of opium poppies and drug abuse in Hebei Province, which seriously hindered local social and economic development. After the founding of the People's Republic of China, Hebei Province launched a large-scale campaign against opium and other drugs. It took the province only about three years to basically eliminate the cultivation, trafficking and consumption of drugs that had lasted for more than a hundred years. The provincial government solved the problem of widespread use of opium and drugs that previous governments had failed to and made the province drugs-free. The success of Hebei's campaign against opium and drugs was mainly attributed to the following factors: attention of government leaders and institutional support, adoption of relevant policies and regulations, public education and people's participation, simultaneously addressing drugs and other social evils, and collaboration among all relevant departments.

Keywords

early years of the People's Republic of China – Hebei Province – campaign against opium and other drugs

Before the founding of the People's Republic of China (PRC) in 1949, exploitative foreign capital and incompetent domestic regimes gave rise to the cultivation of opium poppies and drug abuse in Hebei Province, which seriously

* Dong Xiangqian, Master of Arts in History, works at the Public Foundation Department of Hebei Vocational College of Politics and Law.

 | DOI:10.1163/9789004737990_008

undermined social morality and hindered social and economic development of the province. After opium and other drugs ran rampant in the province, various governments of the province had adopted a strict anti-opium drug policy but failed to solve the problem. In early 1950, shortly after the founding of the PRC, Hebei Province launched a large-scale campaign against opium and drugs. It took the province only about three years to basically eliminate the cultivation, trafficking and consumption of drugs, which had lasted for more than a hundred years. The success of the campaign consolidated the new people's government and brought about profound social changes in Hebei.

1

Opium smoking in Hebei stemmed from the imperialist invasion of the China. About the time of the Opium War in 1840, Western powers' invasion of China brought the import of opium into Hebei (formerly known as Zhili) from Tianjin and other ports. With the import of opium in large quantities, both the nobles and the common people fell into the bad habit of smoking opium. "Most of the military and civilian people as well as current government officials developed the habit."[1] After the Second Opium War, opium trade was legalized and opium became increasingly imported into China from foreign countries. In order to reduce opium imports, the corrupt Qing government adopted the absurd policy of allowing opium poppies to be grown in China, calling it "resisting the foreign with native growth, and using drugs against drugs." After that, opium poppy cultivation began to emerge in Hebei. During Emperor Guangxu's reign of the Qing dynasty, opium poppy cultivation was very popular in Hebei, especially in Qinglong, Weichang and other counties. In 1908, the 34th year of Emperor Guangxu's reign, Cha Meiyin compiled the *Annals of Weichang County*, according to which "The tax levied on opium poppies was 300 coins per *mu*, or 1,700 taels of silver, in the 33rd year of Emperor Guangxu's reign." A calculation based on that would lead to the conclusion that the cultivation area of opium poppies in Weichang County in the year reached as much as 15,700 *mu*.[2] The number of opium addicts multiplied. The Chinese society was in chaos in the early years of the Republic of China. The warlords were in dogfights; opium was rampant; and drugs such as morphine, Trujillo coca, and heroin were prevalent in the province. In 1927, the

1 *Records of Emperor Xuanzong of the Qing Dynasty* (Volume 316).

2 Annals of Hebei Province Compilation Committee, ed. 1993. *Annals of Hebei Province: Public Security*. Beijing: Zhonghua Book Company. 122.

Nationalist government in Nanjing launched a strict anti-opium campaign nationwide, which turned out to be a failure because of corruption within the government and historical limitations. After the Marco Polo Bridge Incident in 1937, the Japanese army invaded and occupied most of Hebei Province and forced local farmers to grow opium poppies. Moreover, they set up an inventory administration and organized drug companies to openly purchase and traffic opium to increase tax revenue. After that, the ban on opium was lifted in Hebei, and the cultivation and production of opium increased sharply. In 1942, more than 100 *mu* of opium poppies were grown in Longfengtai town alone in Changli County.[3] Yangyuan County grew 47,000 *mu* of opium poppies, accounting for 41 percent of the county's arable land, and produced more than 900,000 *liang* of opium annually.[4] Zhangbei County grew opium poppies on half of its arable land.[5] The large-scale cultivation of opium poppies led to a surge in the numbers of opium dens and users. In most cities and counties (and towns) of Hebei, there were points of sale and retail outlets of opium factories where people could buy and smoke opium freely. In addition to opium, other toxic drugs such as heroin and morphine were also flooding the vast areas of Hebei. In the first half of 1946, after Japan's surrender, the Nationalist government of Hebei carried out a province-wide inspection to ban opium smoking, and adopted a joint guarantee policy which connected households and all the connected households would be punished once opium smoking was found in one of them. However, due to the corruption of the government, the campaign against opium and drugs produced limited effect. At the end of the year, more than 1,100 people in the province had quit smoking opium, but the cultivation, production, sale and smoking of opium were still rampant.

In short, opium spread like a virus across Hebei Province in over 100 years from the Opium War to the founding of the PRC and caused damages to almost every town and every village. Countless people lost their family property, had to sell their children with broken families, or even became bandits due to opium-smoking. People's health was seriously damaged; productivity fell sharply; and public interests were severely harmed. During the late Qing dynasty and

3 "Questionnaire on the Losses Caused by Forced Opium Smoking and Cultivation of Opium Poppies During the War of Resistance against Japanese Aggression in Longfengtai Township, Changli County, Hebei Province," in the collection of the Archives of Hebei Province, No.: 615–1-228.

4 Annals of Hebei Province Compilation Committee, ed. 1993. *Annals of Hebei Province: Public Security*. Beijing: Zhonghua Book Company. 123.

5 Public Security Department of the People's Government of Chahar Province. May 23, 1952. "Preliminary Investigation Report on Opium and Other Drugs in Chahar Province," in the collection of the Archives of Hebei Province, No.: 772–1-39.

the Republic of China period, the problem of opium was not solved but became increasingly serious, although the central or local governments organized anti-opium activities,

2

The founding of the PRC on October 1, 1949 opened a new chapter in the history of Hebei Province. The provincial party committee and the provincial government led the people of all ethnic groups in the province to heal the wounds of war, recover the economy, carry out democratic reforms and consolidate the new people's government. The opium-inflicted harm, however, undermined the effort to promote economic recovery and social stability. Therefore, the provincial party committee and the provincial government considered the fight against opium and drugs as an important part of the social reform, and decided to launch an unprecedented campaign against opium and drugs to put an end to the harm that was inflicted by drugs in the past 100 years or more.

In July 1950, in accordance with the Decree on the Prohibition of Opium Drugs issued by the Government Administration Council, the Hebei provincial government issued a directive that it would not purchase opium or allow tax payment in opium instead of grain or the cultivation of opium poppies and that it would launch a large-scale campaign against opium and drugs in the province. The provincial government asked local public security, civil affairs and health departments to take joint actions to close all opium dens, confiscate their houses, smoking utensils and drugs, eradicate opium seedlings, burn all confiscated opium in public, and impose severe criminal penalties on opium producers and dealers and those who had secretly opened opium dens.[6] After the directive was issued, Shijiazhuang, Baoding, Tangshan, Qinhuangdao and other cities of the province set up drug control committees, and some key counties and cities also established drug control offices. All relevant departments worked closely with one another under the same leadership and acted quickly to fulfill their respective responsibilities. Public security departments were responsible for checking trafficking and registration of opium smokers. Health departments were responsible for preparing medicines for helping people quit smoking opium and publicizing their prescriptions, while pharmaceutical manufacturers were responsible for registering and restricting the sale of narcotics. Civil affairs departments were responsible for holding meetings to

6 People's Government of Hebei Province. July 15, 1950. "Reasons for the Prohibition of Opium," in the collection of the Archives of Hebei Province, No.: 907–1-56.

gather information and make plans. The courts were responsible for punishing criminals. People's organizations were responsible for public education. In the course of investigation, they achieved great success in registering opium smokers, inspecting vehicles and ships at stations and customs posts, and encouraging people to report opium smokers and following traces of smokers. For instance, Tangshan cracked down 671 drug cases and seized two hundred *liang* of opium between February 1950 and September 1951.[7] In November 1950, Shijiazhuang burned 266 *liang* of opium and 5.9 *liang* of heroin in public, and organized a public education activity on the spot. The number of opium smokers decreased sharply thanks to compulsory abstinence and education.[8] Chongli County established rehab training teams in Gaojiaying, Xiwanzi, Taipingzhuang and Shizigou that helped more than five hundred well-known serious drug addicts quit drugs through education and labor. Some rehabilitated drug addicts said gratefully: "The Japanese devils turn people into ghosts, and the people's government turns ghosts into people."[9]

To further push forward the campaign and end the harm of drugs, the Hebei provincial government introduced the *Interim Measures on the Prohibition of Opium and Drugs* (the "Measures") in 1951, drawing upon the experience from drug control efforts of 1950. Firstly, the Measures defined the scope of "drugs," including opium, morphine, Trujillo coca, heroin, and other compound substances. Secondly, to ensure smooth progress in drug control, the Measures required people's governments at all levels to set up drug control committees and that civil affairs departments, together with public security, judicial, health and other departments and people's organizations, investigate the cultivation, production, trafficking, sales, smoking or injection of opium and drugs, examine the management of rehab centers, and boost public education to persuade addicts to quit. Thirdly, the Measures specified various policies and specific measures for drug control. The manufacture, trade and trafficking of opium and drugs should be strictly prohibited. The cultivation of opium poppies was forbidden. Privately owned opium should be handed over to the government within a specified time period and the government would provide the owners with compensation to support their lives, but those who failed to do so within the specified time would be punished according to the seriousness of

7 Department of Civil Affairs of the People's Government of Hebei Province. December 24, 1951. "A Report on the Prevalence and Prohibition of Drugs in the Province," in the collection of the Archives of Hebei Province, No.: 937–2-71.

8 Department of Civil Affairs of the People's Government of Hebei Province. December 24, 1951. "A Report on the Prevalence and Prohibition of Drugs in the Province," in the collection of the Archives of Hebei Province, No.: 937–2-71.

9 Zhu Chengming and Guo Yao. "The Harm of Opium." *History of Zhangjiakou* 12: 351.

the case. Drug addicts were required to report to the relevant authorities for registration and to quit using drugs within a time limit, and those who failed to register or did not quit after the time limit would be punished. Fourthly, the Measures also required that cities or regions with high levels of drug use should set up rehab centers and that health authorities at all levels should prepare medicines to help addicts quit using drugs, and reduce fees for poor addicts at their discretion. The Measures fully explained the purpose, principles and policies of drug control, which were applauded by people across the province. Moreover, it also helped to dispel the doubts of many addicts and thus reduce the resistance against drug control. Those actions were of great significance for the smooth advancement of the campaign against opium and drugs. As required by the provincial government, special districts and cities held meetings one after another to make relevant plans and pool resources. Special reconnaissance teams were put together in most areas to challenge the view held by some government officials that there were no drug evils to root out. Thanks to the efforts of the government at all levels and the people, drug control efforts across the province achieved remarkable results. From January 1951 to March 1952, Tangshan Special District cracked down 151 drug cases, of which seventy-one were solved between January and March 1952. Changli, Fuping, and Qianxi counties cracked down eleven to twenty-two cases each, while the number of solved cases was four or five in other counties.[10] Shijiazhuang City found eighty households with major drug-related offences and around two hundred people with minor offences.[11] Tangshan City cracked down seven cases of drug trafficking involving twenty-four thousand *liang* of drugs, including over ten thousand *liang* in one case. In addition, the city found more than fifty households involved in drug-related offences, as well as about five hundred drug addicts and small drug dealers.[12] The campaign against opium and drugs yielded fruitful results and gained a lot of valuable experience, laying a solid foundation for future efforts in this regard.

Hebei's anti-drug campaign of 1950 and 1951 turned out to be a great success. Opium poppy cultivation was basically eliminated in the province; drug

10 June 23, 1952. "The Prevalence of Drugs in Hebei Province and the Plan for Eliminating Drugs," in the archives of the Public Security Department of Hebei Province, File No.: YJ284.

11 June 23, 1952. "The Prevalence of Drugs in Hebei Province and the Plan for Eliminating Drugs," in the archives of the Public Security Department of Hebei Province, File No.: YJ284.

12 June 23, 1952. "The Prevalence of Drugs in Hebei Province and the Plan for Eliminating Drugs," in the archives of the Public Security Department of Hebei Province, File No.: YJ284.

producers and dealers were given a heavy blow; the general public were properly educated; and a large number of drug addicts got rid of their addiction. Given the long history of drug abuse in the province, however, a large amount of privately-owned opium was not confiscated. Some drug dealers were still engaged in illegal activities, and their activities were extremely secretive. Larger drug dealers were mostly in alliances so that they would never give each other away. Some drug users were yet to overcome their addiction. In addition, a few counties were still growing plants for making drugs. According to preliminary statistics in June 1952 on eight cities and districts, such as Tangshan, Shijiazhuang, Qinhuangdao, Baoding, Tongxian and Hengshui, there were still 318 drug dealers, 824 people mostly using drugs and sometimes trafficking drugs, as well as four drug producers.[13] According to incomplete statistics in 1952 on the four special districts of Tongxian, Dingxian, Tianjin and Baoding, 308 villages and 1951 households were growing about 126.4 *mu* of plants for drugs and 67 *mu* of opium poppies.[14] In view of that, drug abuse in Hebei Province remained serious. Therefore, "it is quite necessary to launch a large-scale campaign against drugs across the province with efforts concentrated on important areas."[15]

3

To end the harm of opium and drugs, Hebei Province issued the *Directive on Making Plans for Stopping the Prevalence of Drugs* in April 1952, in accordance with the instructions of the Central Committee of the Communist Party of China (CPC) and its North China Bureau. The Directive pointed out that in light of Hebei's realities, a large-scale people's campaign to stop the prevalence of drugs should be launched, with good preparation, planning and focus, in the later stages of the Three-Anti Campaign (against Corruption, Waste and Bureaucracy) and the Five-Anti Campaign (against Bribery, Tax Evasion, Theft of State Property, Cheating on Government Contracts and Stealing State Economic Information). Hence, the current task to gather all available information, devise plans and make full preparations. In July 1952, Hebei Province

13 June 23, 1952. "The Prevalence of Drugs in Hebei Province and the Plan for Eliminating Drugs," in the archives of the Public Security Department of Hebei Province, File No.: YJ284.

14 June 23, 1952. "Cultivation of Opium and Heroin in Hebei Province," in the archives of the Public Security Department of Hebei Province, File No.: YJ284.

15 June 23, 1952. "The Prevalence of Drugs in Hebei Province and the Plan for Eliminating Drugs," in the archives of the Public Security Department of Hebei Province, File No.: YJ284.

government communicated with local governments the *Directive of the North China Bureau on Making Preparations to Eliminate Drug Use and the Upcoming Briefing Session*, providing more specific instruction on actions to be taken in the preparatory stage. Firstly, clarifying the focus: cities and major transportation routes should be the focus. In-depth investigations and research should be conducted to identify the key areas, key cities, key sectors (e.g. railway, transportation, postal services, telecommunications and customs services), key aspects and key cases. Secondly, available materials should be sorted out and analyzed to find out problems and organize special investigations. Thirdly, reports about drug offenders gathered during the Three-Anti and Five-Anti Campaigns should be examined to check the confessions and clues of the offenders, and the drug offenders released or in prison should be asked questions without letting them know about the real purpose. Fourthly, special networks should be leveraged to penetrate into drug offenders' circles to get hold of ample first-hand information. Fifthly, the experience in dealing with drug offenders should be summed up by calculating the number of drug offenders captured in the past three years and studying the features of their activities. Based on that, proper and effective measures could be devised for future actions. It was made clear that the crackdown policy mainly targeted at drug producers and dealers, instead of drug users who would be educated and transformed later, and that all the drugs already planted must be destroyed. In addition, public security departments at all levels should be responsible for specific operations while other relevant departments should be involved, and all should work in close coordination and collaboration.

Local teams were put together across Hebei to act on the decisions made by the provincial party committee and provincial government. On the one hand, they sorted out available drug-related materials and those collected during the Three-Anti and Five-Anti Campaigns, interrogated the arrested drug offenders, and found out where the drugs came from. On the other hand, they organized educational activities and engaged the general public in a comprehensive investigation into the production, trafficking, transportation and sale of drugs. As of August 7, 1952, 3,653 drug producers and dealers had been found in the province. After further examination, it was found that 1,875 drug offenders remained active after 1951, including thirty-six drug producers and 1,839 drug dealers; twenty-one offenders were from the government sector and 1,854 from non-government sectors. Thorough investigations of 218 cases had been completed or nearly completed.[16]

16 August 7, 1952. "Revised Plan of Hebei Province on Drug Control Action," in the archives of the Public Security Department of Hebei Province, File No.: YJ395.

With full preparation, Hebei Province started a large-scale campaign against drugs from August to October of 1952. In the early stage of the campaign, the provincial government took stock of the cultivation, sale and smoking of opium in the province and listed four cities – Shijiazhuang, Tangshan, Baoding and Qinhuangdao, as well as twenty-six counties and towns including Fuping, Moyuan, Qianxi, Lulong, Changli, Bozhen, Xinji, Shengfang and Yangliuqing as key areas for banning drugs. Railways and transportation departments were designated as major players in the anti-drug campaign.[17] After that, public security, civil affairs, and health departments, courts and other departments worked together in the province-wide people's campaign against drugs. The government of key cities and counties in the province appointed 21,765 communication officials, designated 588 organizers and 9,327 public educators, and held 37,414 public meetings, sub-district office meetings, and industry seminars attended by 2,664,080 persons to educate people on the significance of the campaign against drugs and the harm of drugs to the country and people.[18] They called on people to report and expose cases and traces of drug use, and encouraged drug offenders to turn themselves in and confess to the public security departments. Governments across the province received 39,055 reports and dealt with 3,189 oral reports,[19] indicating the general public were deeply involved in the campaign. The policy for drug users was quite mild. They were mostly encouraged to quit drugs on their own, and there was also supervision and assistance. Except for seniors and patients, all drug addicts were fully rehabilitated. The policy for drug producers and dealers combined severe punishments and reformatory education. The former targeted at the principal offenders, repeated offenders and counter-revolutionaries while the latter at accessory and incidental offenders. At the end of the campaign, governments across the province confiscated 6.81 million *liang* of opium, 3,763 *liang* of opium paste, fifteen *liang* of caffeine sodium benzoate, 3,298 *liang* of caffeine sodium benzoate derivatives, 75.7 *liang* of heroin, as well as 3,216 tools for using drugs, along with fifty-one taels of gold, 924 pieces of silver, twelve million yuan old currency, sixteen pistols and 2,059 bullets.[20] In Zhangbei

17 August 7, 1952. "Revised Plan of Hebei Province on Drug Control Action," in the archives of the Public Security Department of Hebei Province, File No.: YJ395.

18 January 15, 1953. "Implementation of Drug Control Policy," in the archives of the Public Security Department of Hebei Province, File No.: YJ395.

19 1953. "New and Old Administrative Divisions and Drugs in the Province," in the archives of the Public Security Department of Hebei Province, File No.: YJ395.

20 Annals Compilation Committee of Hebei Province, ed. 1993. *Annals of Hebei Province: Public Security*. Beijing: Zhonghua Book Company. 125.

County alone, seventy-two offenders who stocked, sold and used drugs were arrested and punished; twelve were put on public trials, and 257,744 *liang* of opium were confiscated.[21] Apparently, Hebei won a decisive victory in the campaign against drugs.

In brief, Hebei's campaign against opium and drugs from 1950 to 1952 came to an end with an impressive success. The cultivation of opium poppies and the production, sale and use of various drugs were basically eliminated across the province; drug producers and dealers were all severely punished according to the law. It meant that the drugs that had harmed the people of Hebei for more than a century were eliminated three years after the founding of the PRC. Such a success fully showed the superiority of people's democracy and the vitality of the people's government, which greatly enhanced the CPC's prestige among the people of all ethnic groups. It was widely held among the people that "the People's Government had wiped out another great social evil." "In contrast to the CPC's serious drug control, the Nationalist drug control was a sham."[22]

4

It took Hebei only three years to basically eliminate the drugs that had harmed people for over a hundred years. Its success should be attributed to the following factors:

4.1 *Government Leadership and Support*

In the early years of the PRC, most of the leaders of Hebei Province paid much attention to the fight against drugs because they understood the policies of the central government and knew fully well of the harm that drugs had done to the province in the past century. In the course of the fight, leaders at all levels did not just relay the drug control policies of the central government; they instead implemented the policies and regulations in light of the province's realities. Moreover, to ensure smooth progress in the anti-opium campaign, governments at all levels set up drug control committees with representatives from departments of civil affairs, public security, justice and health as well as

21 "The Cultivation, Smoking and Prohibition of Opium in Zhangbei." *History of Zhangjiakou* 22: 223.

22 November 13, 1952. "Summary Report on Drug Control in Hebei Province," in the archives of the Public Security Department of Hebei Province, File No.: YJ227.

people's organizations. The committees were responsible for investigating the cultivation, production, trafficking, sale and consumption of drugs, managing rehab centers, and organizing educational activities to persuade drug addicts to quit smoking. The establishment of drug control committees provided organizational support for the anti-opium campaign. The provincial government also sent working groups to areas with serious drug problems to supervise local drug control efforts and offer guidance and assistance wherever new problems arose. All these contributed substantially to the province's progress in the anti-opium campaign.

4.2 *Adoption of Policies and Regulations*

The provincial government introduced local laws and regulations and specific measures for implementation in light of both the central government's drug control laws and policies and the province's realities. This provided the government officials with applicable laws and policies to follow during the drug control. For example, in view of the fact that too many people were involved in the cultivation and consumption of drugs at the time and the manpower and resources for drug control were rather limited, they adopted the policy banning all drugs with the focus on cracking down on the production and selling drugs to block drug circulation. This proved to be effective because opium poppy growers could not sell the drugs while opium users could not buy what they needed. It was a very successful practice of drug control in the Hebei campaign. In the meantime, feasible and practical measures were adopted to address drug cultivation and consumption. For example, when opium poppy cultivation was banned, poppy growers were encouraged to grow grain and other crops; or they were provided with loans and food to support their life. They also adopted the methods that historically had proved necessary and effective in banning smoking opium, such as registering opium smokers, requiring them to quit within a time limit, helping them quit smoking, etc. All these measures and practices played important roles in advancing the anti-opium campaign.

4.3 *Public Education and People's Participation*

People's participation was another important reason for the rapid success of the anti-opium campaign. Since the spread of drugs was so wide in Hebei, it would be impossible for the government to address the problem without the support and participation of the people. Educational activities helped the people who suffered the most from the drugs to become aware of the harm and get involved in the campaign. Only when they took the initiative to participate could the campaign be successful. In light of that, the provincial government put together special teams to organize educational activities across the province, according to the instruction of the central government. Government officials took the lead with active participants from the general public. Industries and commerce departments, women's federations and many social organizations were fully mobilized as well. Briefing sessions, symposiums, people's meetings, residents' meetings, and meetings of drug dealers' family members were held to ensure the best communication results. Communication teams and vehicles went onto the streets to educate people about the CPC's drug control policy and about the harm of drugs to the mind and body and the development of the PRC. All these made the campaign well known to all people, who became aware that it was illegal to produce and sell opium and harmful to smoke opium. Enlightened people then came forward to report and expose drug offenders. It also exerted strong pressure on drug users, making them feel ashamed. All these helped to ensure the thorough elimination of drugs and the consolidation of achievements in drug control.

4.4 *Addressing Other Social Evils at the Same Time*

In the early years of the PRC, bandits, prostitutes, reactionary cliques and other social evils were as rampant as opium. Some officials in the new government could not change their old mindset, and some even became corrupt, which provided the best soil for the existence or reemergence of opium. Banning opium without cleaning up these social evils would fail to address the problem thoroughly and make it easy for the problem to arise again even when it disappeared for a while. Hebei could achieve the success of the anti-opium campaign and sustained the outcome because it also carried out simultaneously campaigns against bandits, prostitutes, and reactionary guilds during the Three-Anti and Five-Anti Campaigns.

4.5 *Collaboration between Civil Affairs, Public Security, Justice and Health Departments and People's Organizations*

The anti-opium campaign was a complicated project, which required the division of responsibility, coordination, and close collaboration of all relevant departments. In the case of Hebei, public security departments were responsible for checking the trafficking and registration of opium smokers. Health departments were responsible for preparing medicines to help people quit opium-smoking and publicizing the prescriptions, while pharmaceutical manufacturers were responsible for registering and restricting the sale of narcotics. Civil affairs departments were responsible for holding meetings to gather information and make plans. The courts were responsible for punishing criminals. People's organizations were responsible for public education. All these departments worked closely with one another, which played an important role in ensuring the campaign's success.

It was because of these factors that Hebei managed to eliminate the harm of drugs in about three years, improved social morality, restored order, and created a viable social environment for the province to develop politically, economically and culturally.

CHAPTER 8

The Policy of "Uniting Chinese and Western Medicines" in the Early Years of the People's Republic of China

*Tian Gang**

Abstract

In the early years of the People's Republic of China, the policy of "Uniting Chinese and Western Medicines" was introduced at the first National Health Conference. In the process of implementing the policy, however, there emerged a tendency of discriminating against and restricting the practice of Chinese medicine. Mao Zedong and the Central Committee of the Communist Party of China made a timely correction of the mistakes and ensured the full implementation of the policy. The propositions and measures taken by Mao Zedong and the CPC Central Committee in this regard were of great historical and practical significance to the development of Chinese medicine.

Keywords

People's Republic of China – Mao Zedong – "Uniting Chinese and Western Medicines" – health policy

The Communist Party of China (CPC) and the Chinese government have always emphasized the development of healthcare. Sound health policies were introduced in the early years of the People's Republic of China (PRC), which contributed greatly to the improvement of healthcare and people's health. This paper examines the introduction and implementation of the health policy of "Uniting Chinese and Western Medicines" in the early years of the PRC health development and intends to inspire continued efforts of Uniting Chinese and

* Tian Gang is a professor at the School of Health Management and Education, Capital Medical University.

 | DOI:10.1163/9789004737990_009

Western Medicines with a broader perspective of the modernization of traditional Chinese medicine (TCM) and the integration of Chinese and Western medicine.

1 Introduction of the Health Policy of "Uniting Chinese and Western Medicines"

As early as 1928, Mao Zedong proposed, in his article "Struggle in the Jinggang Mountains," a health policy of "utilizing both Chinese and Western medicine for treatment" to solve the problem of treating wounded soldiers during the war.[1] This policy with emphasis on using Chinese medicinal herbs to counter enemy's blockade pointed the direction of combining Chinese medicine with Western medicine in the revolutionary bases. During the War of Resistance Against Japanese Invasion and the War of Liberation, Mao Zedong and the Shaanxi-Gansu-Ningxia Border Region Government repeatedly issued important instructions on how to deal with the traditional medicine of China. In 1940, Mao Zedong stressed the need to unite Chinese and Western medicine and let Chinese medicine play a full role when he attended a conference at the China Medical University to commemorate the anniversary of Dr. Norman Bethune's death. In 1941, the 63rd meeting of the Shaanxi-Gansu-Ningxia Border Region Government emphasized in its resolution on health services that the research on Chinese medicine should be strengthened and the good elements of Chinese medicine be gradually made scientifically.[2] On October 30, 1944, Mao Zedong delivered a speech at the conference of cultural and educational workers in the Shaanxi-Gansu-Ningxia Border Region: "The death rates of people and animals in the region are very high, and many people still believe in witches. In such a situation, it is impossible to solve the problem only by relying on new practitioners of Western medicine. The new doctors are indeed better than the old ones, but if they do not care about the suffering of the people, serve the people, or work with the more than 1,000 traditional doctors and veterinarians in the region and help them to make progress, they are actually helping the witches and watching many people and animals die and doing nothing."[3] Mao

1 Party Literature Research Office of the CPC Central Committee, ed. 1991. *Selected Works of Mao Zedong* (Volume 1). Beijing: People's Publishing House. 65.

2 Li Jingwei. 1986. "The Practice of Traditional Chinese Medicine in China During Revolutionary War." *Journal of Traditional Chinese Medicine* 8.

3 Party Literature Research Office of the CPC Central Committee, ed. 1991. *Selected Works of Mao Zedong* (Volume 3). Beijing: People's Publishing House. 1012.

Zedong once suffered from rheumatoid arthritis and invited Li Dingming, an experienced practitioner of Chinese medicine, to examine him in Yangjialing. When they discussed how to develop Chinese medicine, Li said that Chinese medicine and Western medicine each had their own strengths and that the only way to make progress was to unite them. Mao said, "That's a good idea and we should combine Chinese and Western medicine in the future."[4] This was a reasonable conclusion drawn by Mao Zedong, considering the reality of China and its people and the coexistence of Chinese and Western medicine at the time. This was the earliest evidence of the discussion of Uniting Chinese and Western Medicines. The term and the concept of Uniting Chinese and Western Medicines had been embraced since then, and directly impacted the formation of a series of health policies after the founding of the PRC.

In the early years of the PRC, the high morbidity and mortality rates of various infectious, endemic and occupational diseases caused serious harms to people's health and even reduction of population. Prevention and control of those diseases, therefore, became the most arduous task on the health front. In face of such a situation, Mao Zedong instructed to effectively unite Chinese medicine and to improve it and do a good job in promoting it. Only in this way could the challenging task of protecting the health of hundreds of millions of people be accomplished.[5]

Therefore, after the establishment of the Ministry of Health of the Central People's Government, the first National Health Conference was held in Beijing on August 7, 1950 under the guidance of the CPC Central Committee and Mao Zedong. Mao wrote an inscription for the conference: "Unite all medical practitioners, old and new, Chinese and Western, to form a solid united front for the great cause of protecting the people's health."[6] This instruction by Mao Zedong set the direction of combining Chinese and Western medicine. The conference was presided over by then Health Minister Li Dequan, while Vice Minister He Cheng delivered a report, proposing the three principles of health work as "serving workers, peasants and soldiers; focusing on prevention as the priority; and Uniting Chinese and Western Medicines." They were the major policies guiding the PRC's health construction. In the meantime, four decisions

4 "Doctor Li Dingming Visits Chairman Mao." *Wenhui Daily*, January 16, 1983.

5 Editorial Office of *Series on Contemporary China*, ed. 1986. *Healthcare Sector in Contemporary China* (Volume 2). Beijing: China Social Sciences Press. 69.

6 "Chairman Mao's Inscription for the First National Health Conference." 1978. *Shandong Medical Journal* 12.

on medical education were also announced at the conference, including the decision on the unity and mutual learning of the medical profession.[7]

The three health principles were described in succinct and precise terms. "Serving workers, peasants and soldiers" clearly defined who to be served, indicating the CPC's fundamental purpose of serving the people wholeheartedly and the fact of people being the masters of the country. "Focusing on prevention as the priority" set up the policy and methods of health work by drawing upon the wisdom of working people and the experience of the CPC in developing health services. "Uniting Chinese and Western Medicines" defined the main practice of health services, which became the principle of handling the relations of Chinese and Western medicine – a complicated social problem that had not been properly addressed in modern times. How to treat the hundreds of thousands of practitioners of Chinese medicine in the country and its thousands-year old epistemology was a question that the leaders of the CPC and the Chinese government must consider seriously and address correctly from both political and scientific perspectives. However, some biased views were expressed at the first National Health Conference and by some health professionals which directly affected the implementation of health work.

2 Tendency to Discriminate against and Restrict Chinese Medicine

The Ministry of Health noted in the report delivered at the first National Health Conference that Chinese medicine had accumulated a lot of valuable experience over the past several thousand years, but its theory did not have the foundation of modern science, and that Chinese medicine would not be able to prevent and cure diseases if it stayed the same without changes. "Therefore, efforts should be made to improve Chinese medicine by acquiring political knowledge and modern science, and to combine the experience of TCM with science to make it science-based." "It would require efforts in three aspects to make Chinese medicine science-based. First, the basic knowledge of medical science should be acquired to understand how to manage physiology, anatomy, bacteria, pathology and infectious diseases. Second, TCM practitioners should work with scientists to study Chinese herbal medicine, look into the secret formula, and determine the medicinal properties. Third, Chinese acupuncture should be studied to explore the clinical experience of ancient China and combine it with science. All of those would require the

7 He Cheng. 1951. "Summary Report on the First National Health Conference." *Beijing Journal of Traditional Chinese Medicine* 1.

application of modern scientific knowledge."[8] The scientification of Chinese medicine as proposed in the report would inevitably lead to the Westernization of Chinese medicine. The so-called "science" was nothing but the theories and techniques of Western medicine, and the scientification was to equip TCM practitioners with Western medicine. The health policy of Uniting Chinese and Western Medicines was considered by some leaders at the Health Ministry as an expedient means to ensure political stability and fulfilling the task of disease prevention and treatment. They considered "the united front of Chinese and Western medicine" simply as cooperation in personnel rather than medical knowledge exchange. In 1950, Wang Bin, Vice Minister of Health and Health Director of Northeast China, published an article, "The Organizational Form and Thinking of Healthcare Resulting from the Political and Economic Basis," in *Health in Northeast China* (Volume 1, Issue 9). According to the article, Chinese medicine was born in a feudal society, lacking in scientific knowledge, and could only bring some spiritual comfort to farmers who needed medical treatment; hence, the practice of Chinese medicine should be abolished for the sake of the people. However, "the People's Republic was rather young, it would be impossible to train new doctors equipped with science to replace the TCM practitioners" and "the people would not understand why the practice of Chinese medicine needed to be abolished, given their low level of education and their lack of scientific knowledge." Therefore, "the right policy should not be putting them down," but eliminating them gradually by restrictions.

In a word, the thinking at the first National Health Conference that was embraced by some leaders at the Ministry of Health was to academically transform TCM practitioners and gradually equip them with the theories and techniques of Western medicine, based on the unity and cooperation of Chinese and Western medicine, so that they could serve the cause of people's health. This type of thinking laid the foundation for the formation of TCM policy after the conference.

On May 1, 1951, the Ministry of Health, upon the approval of the Government Administration Council, issued the *Provisional Regulations on TCM Practitioners* (hereinafter referred to as the Regulations), which strictly defined the qualifications of the practitioners.

In term of educational qualifications, the Regulations decided that both the correspondence education and the personal training in Chinese medicine by an experienced practitioner were not to be recognized as meeting the requirements. Only graduates from private or public TCM schools after three to

8 Author unknown. 1950. "Report of the Ministry of Health at the First National Health Conference (Excerpts)." *Journal of New Chinese Medicine* 1(7):6.

four years of training would be issued a TCM practitioner certificate. At that time, however, very few of TCM practitioners, especially the hundreds of thousands of practitioners in rural China, had received formal medical education. Although the certificates issued by the Nationalist government were recognized by the Regulations, very few people had obtained the certificates because the Nationalist government failed to implement the *Regulations on Chinese Medicine* introduced in 1936 after the outbreak of the War Against Japanese Invasion.

According to the Regulations, those who had passed the examinations organized by health authorities at or above the provincial or municipal level and been issued the certificate before the issuance of the Regulations would be eligible for recognition. In reality, however, local authorities were overly strict about the examinations by adopting the principle of "using questions based on science instead of the Chinese medical theories of five *xing* (elements) and six *qi* (vital energy)." According to the appendixes of the *Summary Report on Examinations for Medical Practitioners in Northeast China in 1949*, a total of 2,347 people took the examinations for TCM practitioners and only 173 passed; 128 entered for the examinations on Chinese medicine-based surgery and only eight passed; and 902 took the examinations for TCM pharmacists and only 121 passed.[9]

The Regulations further provided that those who had passed the examinations organized by the Ministry of Health or the health authorities of major administrative regions entrusted by the Central Government would be issued the certificate. However, the *Interim Measures on Examinations for Physicians, TCM Practitioners, Dentists and Pharmacists* was not issued by the Ministry of Health until October 4, 1952. It was impossible that anyone had obtained the TCM certificate before that. The Interim Measures specified the subjects to be covered by the TCM practitioner examination, which included the essentials of Chinese Materia Medica, essentials of ancient formulas, and clinical subjects of Chinese medicine, as well as essentials of physiological anatomy, bacteriology, and infectious diseases (including disinfection methods). All the subjects were obviously too demanding for the TCM practitioners at the time. According to the Regulations and the Interim Measures, there were over fourteen thousand qualified TCM practitioners in 1953 in ninety-two large and medium-sized cities and 165 counties. In Tianjin, a city where Chinese medicine was

9 Deng Guangren. 1955. "The Harm of Wang Bin's Thought in the Archives of the Health Department of Northeast China." *Journal of Traditional Chinese Medicine* 1(8).

better developed, only fifty-five of the more than 530 TCM practitioners who took the examination were qualified.[10]

The Regulations dampened the enthusiasm of a vast number of TCM practitioners. According to statistics, there were five hundred thousand TCM practitioners in early PRC, most of whom were in small towns and rural areas, and over forty thousand in large and medium-sized cities. More than half of urban residents and almost all rural residents relied on TCM practitioners for medical treatment. The implementation of the Regulations led many TCM practitioners to losing their jobs. Some of them shifted to doing business and some became primary school teachers. The loss of TCM practitioners worsened the country's shortage of doctors and medicines.

On December 27, 1951, the Ministry of Health issued the *Regulations on the Organization of Chinese Medicine Schools and Training Classes*, giving clear instructions on the organization, curriculum standards and teaching methods at TCM schools and training classes. The implementation of the Regulations enabled the practicing Chinese doctors to obtain the TCM certificate after they completed studies at a TCM school that was established by the government and passed the graduation examination. However, education at such TCM schools was not intended to produce new TCM practitioners, but to transform the TCM practitioners with the theories and techniques of Western medicine, namely the so-called "scientification of Chinese medicine."

Under the guidance of the aforementioned health policy, it was impossible to produce new TCM practitioners. For the existing TCM practitioners, they had to go through the academic transformation, and those who rejected the transformation or failed in the transformation would be banned from practice. As a result, Chinese medicine was marginalized with heavy losses.

3 Efforts of the CPC Central Committee and Mao Zedong to Correct the Wrong Tendency

During the Three-Anti Campaign including anti-bureaucratism, Mao Zedong read a report written by Bai Xueguang about the bureaucratic style of the Health Department of the Military Commission. On April 3, 1953, Mao sent an instruction: "Comrades Zhou Enlai, Xi Zhongxun, Hu Qiaomu, Peng Dehuai, Huang Kecheng and He Cheng: The report by Bai Xueguang exposed the extremely serious bureaucracy among the leaders of the Military Commission's Health

10 Department of Traditional Chinese Medicine, Ministry of Health of China. 1985. *A Collection of Documents on Traditional Chinese Medicine (1949–1983)*. 38–39, 216.

Department ... This reminds me of the need to check if the Ministry of Health has the same problem. I suspect that the leadership of the Ministry of Health is performing as badly as the leadership of the Military Commission's Health Department, offering neither political guidance nor careful professional and technical leadership. If it were not for Bai Xueguang's detailed exposure, we wouldn't know the real situation. Please Xi and Qiao, go and inspect carefully the work at the Ministry of Health, by using Bai Xueguang's report as the reference, to see if they are doing any better than the Military Commission's Health Department? Find out solutions to any problems identified and put them into practice. There are probably other bureaucratic departments like the Military Commission's Health Department, which offered no leadership, no political guidance and no good professional management but only have their meals (get salaries) and occupy official positions as if they were the masters. I ask you to be bold and resolute, standing no ceremony, in the fight against bureaucratism and to transform them into government agencies that can do the work."[11]

Following Mao's instructions, the Culture and Education Committee of the Central Government Administration Council conducted an in-depth inspection of the work at the Ministry of Health. They found that the Ministry of Health had made serious mistakes in implementing the health policy of "Uniting Chinese and Western Medicines" by discriminating and restricting the practice of Chinese medicine. Therefore, Mao Zedong made several speeches and instructions around the Spring Festival in 1954, emphasizing the need to improve the work of Chinese medicine and implement the combination of Chinese and Western medicine. All these provided the guidance for the health authorities to formulate correct policy regarding Chinese medicine.

On February 25, 1954, the 206th Meeting of the Government Administration Council approved the resolution adopted by the Third National Health Administration Conference. In taking stock of the work done by the Ministry of Health in the past four years, the resolution pointed out: "We are often biased by focusing on the shortcomings of Chinese medicine and fail to see it as part of China's valuable cultural heritage that plays an important role among the people. As a result, Chinese medicine has been neglected and discriminated against."[12] The resolution stressed that a series of measures must be taken to promote Chinese medicine and let it play the full role in society. The resolution

---

11 Party Literature Research Office of the CPC Central Committee, ed.1990. *Manuscripts of Mao Zedong Since the Founding of the People's Republic of China* (Volume 4). Beijing: Central Party Literature Publishing House. 176–177.

12 Author unknown. 1994. "Resolution of the Third National Health Administrative Conference." *Journal of New Chinese Medicine* 5 (8):233.

basically embodied Mao's instruction about improving the work on Chinese medicine.

On July 9, 1954, Liu Shaoqi conveyed Mao Zedong's new instructions on the issue of Chinese medicine to the Party Leadership Group of the Central Cultural Affairs Commission. On July 12, the Central Cultural Affairs Commission held an enlarged meeting of its Party Leadership Group to communicate and discuss the instructions. The meeting decided that under the leadership of the Party Leadership Group, a temporary working group on Chinese medicine would be formed by the Central Publicity Department, the Central Cultural Affairs Commission and the Ministry of Health to conduct investigations and research. On October 26, the Party Leadership Group submitted the *Report to the CPC Central Committee on Improving the Work of Chinese Medicine*.

The report pointed out that it was a good thing that Western medicine had widely spread in China since the late 19th and early 20th century. But along with it came the misleading notion and attitude that Western medicine was absolutely all good and that Chinese medicine was backward and had no merit at all. As a result, there developed an arrogant and contemptuous attitude toward Chinese medicine, which caused the exclusion of Chinese medicine and the hostile relations between Chinese and Western medicine. It was not a surprise that the attitude existed in the old semi-colonial China. "The serious problem is that this kind of hostility and sectarianism against Chinese medicine was not criticized or corrected but grew after the founding of the PRC."[13] For a few years, the Ministry of Health did some work about Chinese medicine and made some achievements, but the policy of Uniting Chinese and Western Medicines was not well implemented in its overall thinking. To change this situation, the report recommended the establishment of a Chinese Medicine Academy, accepting TCM practitioners to work at large hospitals, expanding and improving Chinese medicine services, and improving TCM practitioners' training. It further recommended better management of the production and marketing of Chinese herbal medicine, publishing Chinese medicine books, and accepting TCM practitioners as members of the Chinese Medical Association to make it a people's academic organization in the country's medical community. The report was approved by the Central Government on November 23, and the implementation of the recommendations played a very important role in promoting the development of Chinese medicine.

After discovering the wrong tendency of the Ministry of Health in discriminating against and restricting Chinese medicine, Mao Zedong paid more

13 Department of Traditional Chinese Medicine, Ministry of Health of China. 1985. *A Collection of Documents on Traditional Chinese Medicine (1949–1983)*. 42.

attention to Chinese medicine. He made a series of publications which helped promote the development of Chinese medicine, and also provide us with valuable inspirations today.[14]

3.1 *Mao Zedong Explained the Scientific Nature of Chinese Medicine and Its Great Contribution in the History of China, Noting That "Chinese Medicine Is a Great Treasure House"*

Those who discriminated against and opposed Chinese medicine often used the knowledge of modern natural science and Western medicine in simple comparison to attack it as superstitious, false and unscientific. Mao Zedong was keenly aware of this mistake and resolutely opposed the use of Western medical theories to measure the scientific nature of Chinese medical theories. He said: "Practice is the sole criterion for testing the truth. Some principles of Chinese medicine may not be easy to understand but have proved to be effective. This is what truth is about."[15] It is about what actually happened in reality. In ancient times, people tried to understand the human body through direct observations of the sensory organs, and explained the unknown by making analogies of the known. They managed to understand the essence of things by observing the outside to understand the inside. They observed the functional structure and innate connections of the human body as a whole and came to understand some of the mysteries of human life and the patterns of diseases. The Chinese medicine theories that were established have proved effective in disease prevention and treatment. The reason that Chinese medicine can last so long with vitality precisely because it has produced effective therapeutic methods. Therefore, Mao Zedong said, "China is the most populous country in the world. There are many reasons why the Chinese nation has been thriving with a large population. Healthcare is surely one of the important reasons, and the first credit should be given to Chinese medicine."[16] From this point of view, the contribution of Chinse medicine is indeed much greater than that of Western medicine. "In comparison, Chinese medicine has a history of several thousand years, while Western medicine has been around only for about one hundred years since its introduction to China ... Therefore, in regard to the history of China's healthcare, the contributions and accomplishments of

14 Wang Hongjie. 2002. "A Study of Mao Zedong's Thoughts on the Culture of Traditional Chinese Medicine." Master's Thesis of Shanghai Jiao Tong University.

15 Ma Boying. 1993. *The History of Intercultural Medicine Communication Between China and Foreign Countries*. Shanghai: Wenhui Publishing House. 547.

16 Ma Boying. 1993. *The History of Intercultural Medicine Communication Between China and Foreign Countries*. Shanghai: Wenhui Publishing House. 577.

Chinese medicine are substantial, while that of Western medicine is relatively insignificant."[17] We have no justification to negate Chinese medicine. "Chinese medicine has developed by drawing on lessons learned from Chinese people's fight against diseases in the past thousands of years. It contains the rich experiences and theoretical knowledge of Chinese people fighting against diseases. It is a great treasure house."[18]

3.2 *Mao Zedong Encouraged the Exploration and Continuous Use of the Medical Heritage of Ancient China*

When the PRC was founded, it faced the challenges of a collapsed economy and the difficult task of reconstruction. The exhausting demand for healthcare required the urgent collaboration of Chinese and Western medicine to work together and play their respective roles in serving the people. Therefore, Mao Zedong wrote an inscription for the first National Health Conference that read "Unite all medical practitioners, old and new, Chinese and Western, to form a solid united front for the great cause of protecting the people's health."[19] Mao firmly criticized the mistakes of discriminating against and restricting Chinese medicine. He repeatedly emphasized the need to study and promote Chinese medicine, for fear that "this part of China's cultural heritage would be in danger of being lost, which is absolutely not acceptable."[20] Modern methods, that is, scientific principles, should be used to study Chinese medicine and Chinese herbal medicine. "We must learn the principles of science from foreign countries and then apply them to the study of Chinese things."[21] In response to the tendency of organizing TCM practitioners to study Western medicine and to transform them with Western medicine, Mao Zedong creatively emphasized the importance of organizing practitioners of Western medicine to study Chinese medicine and put forward the idea that "the first step should be practitioners of Western medicine studying Chinese medicine, rather than TCM

17 Ma Boying. 1993. *The History of Intercultural Medicine Communication Between China and Foreign Countries*. Shanghai: Wenhui Publishing House. 577.

18 Party Literature Research Office of the CPC Central Committee, ed. 2003. *Selected Letters of Mao Zedong*. Beijing: Central Party Literature Publishing House. 503.

19 Author unknown. "Chairman Mao's Inscription for the First National Health Conference." 1978. *Shandong Medical Journal* 12.

20 National Administration of Traditional Chinese Medicine. 1990. *A Collection of Documents on Traditional Chinese Medicine*. Beijing: China Medical Science and Technology Press. 43.

21 Mao Zedong. "A Talk with Musicians (August 24, 1956)." *The People's Daily*, September 9, 1979.

practitioners studying Western medicine."[22] Mao also personally inspected health work and extensively solicited opinions of the TCM community. He proposed specific measures to improve Chinese medicine: First, choose one hundred to two hundred medical college graduates and sent them to famous TCM practitioners to learn from their clinical experience. High-level research institutes of Chinese medicine should be established to study Chinese medicine, with participation of both famous TCM practitioners and practitioners of Western medicine who had basic knowledge of Chinese medicine. Second, hospitals should have a plan of inviting TCM practitioners to see patients with diagnosis and treatment, allow in-patients to use Chinese herbal medicine, and hammer out the rules of respecting TCM practitioners. Third, protect and develop Chinese herbal medicine. The study of Chinese herbal medicine should include not only chemical analysis but also pharmaceutical testing and clinical trials, especially the synergy of Chinese herbal medicine. Fourth, sort out the books of Chinese medicine and organize scholars of Chinese medicine to translate some useful ancient TCM books into modern texts with a plan and concentration. When the time comes, they should be called to come together to sort out their experience and compile systematically a full set of Chinese medicine books.[23] Those measures emphasized on carrying forward Chinese medicine culture and reflected what TCM practitioners wanted. Their implementation significantly contributed to the development of Chinese medicine and pharmacology.

3.3 *Mao Zedong Proposed the Important Goal of Combining Chinese and Western Medicine to Create a New Integrated Medical and Pharmaceutical Science in China*

Mao Zedong's thought on combining Chinese and Western medicine aimed at creating a new medical and pharmaceutical science in China. He clearly pointed out at the Political Bureau's meeting in 1953: "Chinese medicine and Western medicine must unite and work together. Western medicine must break its sectarianism. There will be only one medicine and not two medicines; the one medicine must be guided by materialistic dialectics."[24] In a talk with writers and artists in 1956, Mao further specified that "the knowledge

22 Ma Boying. 1993. *The History of Intercultural Medicine Communication Between China and Foreign Countries*. Shanghai: Wenhui Publishing House. 577.

23 Xing Sishao. "Mao Zedong's Attention to the Cause of Traditional Chinese Medicine." *Health News*, December 15, 1983.

24 Ma Boying. 1993. *The History of Intercultural Medicine Communication Between China and Foreign Countries*. Shanghai: Wenhui Publishing House. 545.

of Chinese medicine and pharmacology should be combined with that of Western medicine and pharmacology to create a new integrated medical and pharmaceutical science in China."[25]

Chinese and Western medicine should be combined because they both study the same thing – human diseases and health, and they both offer the theories on human life, aging, illness and death. They are of the same discipline of studies, according to Mao's classification of academic disciplines by their specialties. Mao further detailed: "The distinction of scientific research is based on the particularity of research subjects. Therefore, a certain phenomenon peculiar to a certain field constitutes the subject matter of a certain science."[26] There is only one medical science. Chinese medicine and Western medicine are not two separate medical disciplines, but two schools of thought in the same discipline. Chinese medicine and Western medicine have observed and studied the same subjects from their respective angles, and have gained insights into different laws of life and health or different sides of the same law. Therefore, they differ widely in the content, approach and model of academic studies. They each have their limitations and strengths in their understandings of the human body. Mao Zedong believed that there was no such thing as commonality or particularity between different nations when it came to scientific principles. "Every field of study is about the basic theories, which is the same in China and other countries. They should not be separated with the label Chinese or Western. All countries agree on, for example, what makes water and humans are descended from apes." Other issues that do not distinguish one nation from another include appendectomy and taking aspirin, Chinese angelica, rhubarb, etc. to cure diseases. Therefore, Mao Zedong emphasized that "We need to make it very clear: we must learn from the West, as far as the fundamental principles are concerned. It does not make sense that the scalpel has to be Chinese."[27] Mao Zedong's argument is indeed insightful. The basic patterns of diseases are fundamentally consistent in Chinese medicine and Western medicine. The cellular pathology discovered by Western medicine applies to Chinese people, while the meridians discovered by Chinese medicine apply to peoples of other countries in the world. The same research subjects of Chinese medicine and Western medicine determine the feasibility of combining

25 "Vigorously Accelerating the Development of Traditional Chinese Medicine." *The People's Daily*, November 2, 1978.

26 Party Literature Research Office of the CPC Central Committee, ed. 1991. *Selected Works of Mao Zedong* (Volume 1). Beijing: People's Publishing House. 309.

27 Mao Zedong. "A Talk with Musicians (August 24, 1956)." *The People's Daily*, September 9, 1979.

Chinese and Western medicine, whereas the limitations of both Chinese and Western medicine make it necessary to combine the two. They will make new inventions when the two combine. In fact, it is not enough to overcome the limitations of either Western medicine or Chinese medicine when Western medicine draws upon some advantages of Chinese medicine or Chinese medicine draws upon some advantages of Western medicine. They only add a few new things to the existing theories of Western or Chinese medicine. Mao Zedong had always stressed the need to "combine Chinese and foreign theories organically."[28] The new medical and pharmaceutical sciences formed through the combination of Chinese and Western medicine will overcome their limitations and delve deeper in the exploration of health and disease to push the understanding of life to a new level. Such a new medical theory system, based on but better than Chinese medicine and Western medicine, is exactly what Mao Zedong had hoped for.

4 The Significance of Correctly Upholding the Health Policy of "Uniting Chinese and Western Medicines"

4.1 *Directly Promoting the Development of Chinese Medicine*

In 1954, meetings and forums of the representatives of Chinese medicine were held in places such as the East China Region, Shanghai, Tianjin, Sichuan, Xikang and Shaanxi to discuss how to organize and exert the power of Chinese medicine, sort out the academic works of Chinese medicine, and advance the studies of Chinese medicine. The Chinese Medical Association (CMA) issued the instruction to promote Chinese medicine. It noted that Chinese medicine was an integral part of Chinese cultural heritage and that the majority of Chinese people relied on Chinese medicine for treatment of illnesses. The promotion of Chinese medicine was a serious matter that concerned the health of Chinese people.[29] In November of the same year, the Ministry of Health established the Department of Chinese Medicine. On December 12, 1955, the China Academy of Chinese Medicine was established. Premier Zhou Enlai wrote an inscription for the academy, which read "To Carry Forward Our Medical Heritage and to Serve the Construction of Socialism."[30] In 1956, the

28 Mao Zedong. "A Talk with Musicians (August 24, 1956)." *The People's Daily*, September 9, 1979.

29 "Chinese Medical Association Issues a Directive to Promote the Practice of TCM." *The People's Daily*, October 22, 1954.

30 See the cover of *Journal of New Chinese Medicine*, January 1956.

Ministry of Health ordered the cancellation of four documents that had hindered the development of Chinese medicine, including the *Provisional Regulations on Traditional Chinese Medicine Practitioners* and the *Interim Measures for the Examinations of Traditional Chinese Medicine Practitioners*. It stressed the implementation of the policy of Uniting Chinese and Western Medicines and developing Chinese medicine. When the China Academy of Chinese Medical Sciences was established, the first Chinese medicine training program for Western medicine practitioners started, bringing together 76 experienced doctors of Western medicine from across the country. They took leave of their jobs and received training in Chinese medicine for two and a half years with great results. On November 18, 1958, the CPC Central Committee approved the *Summary Report on the Off-the-job Chinese Medicine Training Program for Western Medicine Practitioners* submitted by the party leadership of the Ministry of Health. It confirmed the training and noted that "there might emerge some great theorists among them and it should not be taken lightly."[31] Most of the trainees later became the leading scientists or top professionals in Chinese medicine or in combining Chinese and Western medicine. Thanks to such efforts, the number of Western medicine practitioners studying Chinese medicine increased significantly across the country. According to the statistics of 1960, about thirty-six thousand Western medicine doctors received on-the-job training in Chinse medicine across the country, and a number of students showed keen interest in studying Chinese medicine at many medical and pharmacy colleges and schools.[32]

Shortly after its establishment, the China Academy of Chinese Medicine organized experts to sort out Chinese medicine books and compile Chinese medicine textbooks in nine categories. These books became important references for Western medicine to learn Chinese medicine and for the education of Chinese medicine. Furthermore, the Ministry of Health organized five medical colleges of Chinese medicine in Beijing, Shanghai, Guangzhou and other cities in 1960 to compile *Lectures on Chinese Medical History*, *Lectures on Ancient Medical Texts*, *Lectures on the Diagnostics of Chinese Medicine*, *Lectures on Chinese Pharmacology*, *Lectures on the Formulas of Chinese Medicine*, *Lectures on Chinese Internal Medicine*, *Lectures on Acupuncture and Moxibustion*, *Lectures on the Gynecology of Chinese Medicine*, and *Lectures on the Pediatrics*

---

31 Party Literature Research Office of the CPC Central Committee, ed. 1995. *Selected Important Documents Since the Founding of the People's Republic of China* (Volume 11). Beijing: Central Party Literature Publishing House. 566–567.

32 Department of Traditional Chinese Medicine, Ministry of Health of China. 1985. *A Collection of Documents on Traditional Chinese Medicine (1949–1983)*. 173.

of Chinese Medicine.[33] In the meantime, the Ministry of Health assigned scientific research tasks through national competitive bidding to sort out and revise ancient Chinese medical books. The publication of many ancient medical books facilitated the training of high-level specialized talents with complete mastery of Chinese medicine theories and clinical skills. All those measures promoted the rapid development of Chinese medicine.

4.2 *Providing the Theoretical and Practical Basis for the Development of Chinese Medicine in the New Era*

The Chinese medicine enterprise initiated by the first generation of the central leadership with Mao Zedong at its core has been inherited and carried forward well. In September 1978, the CPC Central Committee forwarded to relevant agencies the report by the Party Leadership Group of the Ministry of Health, "On Firmly Implementing the Party's Chinese Medicine Policy and Addressing the Problem of the Shortage of Young Chinese Medicine Practitioners." The Committee emphasized in the comments that the shortage of young TCM practitioners was an urgent matter that needed to be addressed fast by developing a high-level contingent of TCM practitioners proficient in theories and rich in clinical experience and by creating a team of Western medicine doctors who are enthusiastic about studying TCM and combining Chinese and Western medicine. In his instruction, Deng Xiaoping pointed out specifically, "This issue should be taken seriously, and in particular, we must create favorable material conditions for the development and improvement of Chinese medicine."[34]

The central government adopted special measures and policies to restore the administrative organizations and various specialized colleges to revitalize Chinese medicine. "The development of modern medicine and China's traditional medicine" was written into the newly revised constitution. The central government introduced a number of policies and regulations to preserve and develop Chinese medicine and culture. An outline for the development of Chinese Medicine was created for the period of 1988–2000. China upheld the open-up policy and developed cooperation with more countries and regions in the world in the field of traditional medicine.

---

33 Li Jingwei. 2006. *History of Thoughts on Traditional Chinese Medicine*. Changsha: Hunan Education Publishing House. 732.

34 Author unknown. 2004. "Deng Xiaoping's Instructions on the Practice of Traditional Chinese Medicine – Commemorating the 100th Birthday of Deng Xiaoping." *Jiangsu Journal of Traditional Chinese Medicine* 9.

While advancing the cause of building socialism with Chinese characteristics into the 21st century, Jiang Zemin and the CPC Central Committee used the Three Represents Theory as guidance, followed the cultural program of the primary stage of socialism, and proceeded from the perspective of developing an advanced socialist culture and innovative theory. They summed up past experiences and lessons and pointed out: "Chinese medicine is a special feature of Chinese medical science and an important part of the outstanding Chinese culture. It has contributed to the development of Chinese civilization and exerted a positive influence on the progress of world civilization. We should correctly handle the relationship between its inheritance and its development to promote its modernization. Chinese medicine and Western medicine are equally important and they should be developed together to complement each other so as to provide people with better and more effective healthcare services."[35] To implement the directive of the CPC Central Committee on "strengthening Chinese medicine research and revitalizing Chinese medicine,"[36] relevant departments adopted a series of measures, such as stressing the need to study and develop Mao Zedong's thoughts on Chinese medicine, summing up the successful achievements in combining Chinese and Western medicine, realizing the modernization of Chinese medicine, keeping "the equal importance of Chinese and Western medicine" as the basic health policy in the new era, revising and improving the laws and regulations on Chinese medicine, strengthening the reform and development of healthcare, establishing new administrative organizations and educational institutions of Chinese medicine, creating the "Ten-Year Plan for International Exchange and Cooperation on Chinese Medicine," and promoting international exchanges and cooperation of Chinese medicine.

At present, the CPC Central Committee, with Hu Jintao as the General Secretary, pays great attention to the development of Chinese medicine and stresses the equal importance of Chinse and Western medicine in the development of Chinese medicine and the nation's medicine in order to build a harmonious socialist society and an innovative country.[37] "The Outline Plan for the Innovative Development of Chinese Medicine (2006–2020)" has been

35 "National Administration of Traditional Chinese Medicine Holds an Experts' Seminar to Learn the Guidelines of General Secretary Jiang's Speech on the Practice of Traditional Chinese Medicine." *Guangming Daily*, March 19, 2001.

36 See the cover of 1993. *Journal of Traditional Chinese Medicine Management* 1.

37 Hu Jintao. "Hold High the Great Banner of Socialism with Chinese Characteristics and Strive for New Victories in Building a Moderately Prosperous Society in all Respects: Report to the Seventeenth National Congress of the Communist Party of China." *The People's Daily*, October 25, 2007.

unveiled with comprehensive arrangements for the development of Chinese medicine. They include a guideline that defines "the full use of modern science and technology to prove the scientific nature of Chinese medicine on the basis of promoting its unique strengths, to improve TCM service capacity and the technological content of Chinese herbal medicine industry through technological innovation, and to enhance and improve TCM theoretical system and healthcare model through knowledge innovation." The basic principle was to "give equal emphasis to inheritance and innovation, to promote the coordinated development of TCM and Chinese herbal medicine, to draw upon modern and international elements, and to combine multiple disciplines." Efforts should be made to improve the technical system of Chinese medicine in disease prevention, health preservation, and diagnosis and treatment, complete the modern industrial system for Chinese herbal medicine, develop the theoretical system of Chinese medicine, establish an internationally recognized standard system for Chinese medicine, build a scientific and technological innovation system fit for the characteristics of Chinese medicine, and form an international scientific and technological cooperation network." The ultimate purpose is to "promote the complementarity and integration of Chinese and Western medicine to lay the foundation for a new medicine with Chinese characteristics."[38] The CPC has been consistent in protecting and developing Chinese medicine and culture, starting from Mao Zedong's idea of "combining Chinese and Western medicine to create a new medical and pharmaceutical science in China" to the policy of "promoting the complementarity and integration of Chinese and Western medicine to lay the foundation for a new medicine with Chinese characteristics."

4.3 *Mao Zedong's Thought of Combining Chinese and Western Medicine Opened Up a New Path for Medical Development in China*

The important propositions of Mao Zedong, such as "Chinese medicine is a great treasure house that should be explored and improved" and "the knowledge of Chinese medicine should be combined with that of Western medicine to create a new medical and pharmaceutical science in China," have been gradually understood by medical professionals and shared by the majority of people. Under the guidance of such policies, practitioners of Western medicine have sought to learn from experienced TCM practitioners with an open mind and drawn upon their clinical experience for improvement. As a result,

38 Liu Shu. "Interpretation of the Outline of the Plan for Innovative Development of Traditional Chinese Medicine." *Science and Technology Daily*, March 21, 2007.

thousands of senior doctors with expertise in both Chinese and Western medicine have emerged, including a number of experts well known in China and other countries. The combination of Chinese and Western medicine has provided an effective way to prevent and cure diseases and raise the level of medical services. It helped the development of basic TCM theories, expanded the dialectical connotations, and enriched the content of modern medicine. It has also expanded the application scope of TCM, promoted the research and development of new Chinese herbal medicine and the improvement of TCM formulas, and facilitated international academic exchanges and cooperation in TCM research. Other countries have become interested in acupuncture and acupuncture anesthesia because of the research on combining Chinese and Western medicine. Now, the work of combining Chinese and Western medicine has gone beyond China as a global scientific endeavor.

4.4 *The Practice of Combining Chinese and Western Medicine Inspired Other Countries and Regions to Address Their Traditional Medicines*

In the past two hundred years, Western medicine has grown rapidly and practiced all over the world. The traditional medicines indigenous in many countries and regions have lost their legitimacy under the impact of Western medicine. Traditional Chinese medicine, however, has been able to last for a long time and shown great vitality. It suggests that Chinese medicine contains scientific essence and strong vitality, while at the same time, its development is inseparable from Mao Zedong's vision and the support of the government. The PRC cherishes the development of national cultural heritage. It has adopted the policy of protecting and supporting Chinese medicine, making China the only country in the world where two kinds of medicine coexist. On the basis of mutual learning, practitioners of Chinese and Western medicine have conducted collaborative research according to national plan and made a host of remarkable clinical achievements. The achievements of Chinese medicine have drawn attention from around the world. Some countries and regions have been encouraged by the TCM achievements to re-examine their traditional medicines. Inspired by the Chinese government's efforts to protect and develop TCM, the World Health Organization (WHO) has increased its attention to traditional medicine in recent years. In November 1997, it held a conference on the promotion and development of traditional medicine in Geneva. The conference report noted that traditional medicine had proved to be effective and practical, and that it should be formally recognized and promoted. In May 1998, the World Health Assembly adopted the "Resolution on the Promotion and Development of the Training and Research in Traditional Medicine," according to which a committee of traditional medical experts was to be established in WHO to take charge of holding international conferences, communicating information, developing talents, and carrying out multidisciplinary research. The research of traditional medicine in many countries began to develop, thanks to the efforts of WHO.

Today, as we face many challenges in the endeavor to modernize TCM and promote the integration of Chinese and Western medicine, a review of the Chinese history of medicine shows that Mao Zedong's assessment of the TCM's value is objective and the policy of Uniting Chinese and Western Medicines formed in the early years of the PRC is correct and in line with the objective laws of science. We must uphold the thought of combining Chinese and Western medicine and advance the work of modernizing Chinese medicine and the cause of combining Chinese and Western medicine with a broader vision and from a higher starting point.

CHAPTER 9

China's Patriotic Hygiene Campaign, 1949–1959

*Xiao Aishu**

Abstract

From 1949 to 1959, the Communist Party of China (CPC) and the Chinese government conducted a nationwide Patriotic Hygiene Campaign which achieved the desired outcomes. This campaign not only improved the health of the Chinese people and played an important role in promoting good habits but also fully demonstrated the superiority of people's democracy and the tremendous power exerted by the people under this system. This campaign informed policymakers and provided good practices in public health.

Keywords

People's Republic of China – the Four Pests Campaign – Patriotic Hygiene Campaign

After the founding of the People's Republic of China, under the leadership of the CPC and the people's governments at all levels, Chinese people actively participated in the War to Resist the U.S. Aggression and Aid Korea, suppression of counter-revolutionaries, the Land Reform, the movements against "three evils" and "five evils", the Cooperative Movement, and the Patriotic Hygiene Campaign. The Patriotic Hygiene Campaign not only improved access to sanitation in urban and rural areas and people's ability to fight diseases but also fully demonstrated the superiority of people's democracy and the tremendous power exerted by the people under this system. It informed policymakers and provided good practices in public health.

* Xiao Aishu, born in 1954, associate professor and Ph.D. Candidate at the History Department of Jining Normal University, and Department of History of Nanjing University.

 | DOI:10.1163/9789004737990_010

1

Public health promotes and protects the health of people. It is vital to maintain a strong workforce for the country. In the early days of the PRC, the country's healthcare sector focused on serving workers, peasants and soldiers, prioritizing prevention and integrating Chinese and Western medicine. In the initial stage of the Patriotic Hygiene Campaign, the country focused on controlling the deadliest infectious diseases, especially smallpox, plague, and cholera, which threatened national security. According to the *Comprehensive Report on Epidemic Prevention in the Past 21 Months* submitted by the Vice Minister of Health He Cheng to the CPC Central Committee in September 1951, over 17,000 Chinese citizens had been vaccinated against smallpox using the cowpox vaccine in less than two years since the founding of the People's Republic of China. In areas such as Northeast China, Inner Mongolia, Hebei, Jiangxi, Shaanxi, Fujian, Tianjin, and Wuhan, smallpox cases in 1951 decreased by more than half compared with 1950. No smallpox case had been reported in the two years in Lǚda, Yingkou, Qinhuangdao, Yantai, Xiamen, Guangzhou, Beijing and other cities, to control the spread of the plague, health departments set up plague control stations in eight areas severely hit by the plague, mobilizing the masses to exterminate rats and fleas and get vaccinated.

In 1951, the plague in Inner Mongolia, Northeast China, and Chahar was effectively controlled, and the number of plague cases in the country from January to June decreased by 78 per cent compared with the same period in 1950. The cure rate of patients with plague increased by 17 per cent compared with 1950. Cholera had broken out in the country every year since it made its way to China in 1820. China strengthened quarantine measures to prevent cross-border transmission of cholera and stepped up inspections to ensure patients would be identified as soon as possible. It also attached great importance to drinking water disinfection, sanitation, and vaccination. Due to the above measures, no classic cholera patient was found after the founding of the People's Republic of China.[1] To use the epidemic prevention resources flexibly, the Ministry of Health dispatched 125 epidemic prevention teams (6,000 health workers) to areas affected by disasters or epidemics. The areas covered by the Huaihe River Project engaged the general public in a large-scale

1 Gao Enxian. 2000. "Documents on Healthcare Approved by Mao Zedong in the Early Days of the Founding of the People's Republic of China." *Journal of Chinese Medical History* 1: 45–46.

sanitation and epidemic prevention campaign, effectively controlling the spread of typhus, relapsing fever, typhoid fever, and dysentery.[2]

The country also achieved remarkable results in preventing the spread of other infectious diseases, such as kala-azar, venereal disease, and malaria. The Ministry of Health set up eight specialized healthcare centers for control of kala-azar, which was prevalent on both banks of the Yellow River and along the Longhai Railway. These centers cured more than 110,000 patients in two years. In 1951, BHC powder was sprayed in the areas mentioned above, leading to a significant drop in the reproduction of sand flies, which can transmit the infectious pathogen and kill the dogs infected with the disease. These measures effectively reduced the number of patients with kala-azar in northern Jiangsu and other areas. To control the spread of schistosomiasis, 18 control centers or stations were set up in the Yangtze River Basin to conduct experiments and kill Oncomelania that can cause the disease. A three-cylinder fecal storage method was advocated to kill parasites and their eggs in the feces. To control tuberculosis, 850,000 children in 82 cities were vaccinated with BCG. In Beijing, Suiyuan, and Xi'an, women who used to be prostitutes received treatment for STDs. The country also strengthened STD prevention in ethnic minority communities. The health department of Inner Mongolia has strengthened STD prevention efforts in every banner since 1950, and the fertility rate in Chenba'erhu Banner rose fast. According to the resolution of the second meeting of the Chinese People's Political Consultative Conference (CPPCC), the Ministry of Health dispatched the 7th Brigade of the Central Infectious Disease Prevention and Control Corps to treat 120,000 patients with STDs in the ethnic Tibetan and Mongolian communities in Gansu and Qinghai. A medical team composed of professors and students of Peking University Medical School visited Suimeng and Inner Mongolia to assist in STD prevention during the summer vacations of two consecutive years. The country also attached great importance to the prevention and control of infectious diseases in kids, for example, the mortality rate of patients with measles used to be very high in China. In 1951, thanks to strengthened publicity and prevention efforts, the mortality rate dropped from 8.5 per cent in the previous year to 5 per cent.[3]

The Ministry of Health convened the National Infectious Disease Prevention and Control Conference in April 1951 to summarize work it had done since the

2 Li Dequan. "Strive to Further Improve Public Health. *Xinhua Monthly*." November 1951, 37.

3 Li Dequan. "Report on National Disease Prevention and Control." *The People's Daily*, January 11, 1952.

founding of the People's Republic of China and formulate a work plan. While affirming past achievements, it reviewed its deficiencies in the following areas:

1. It focused on acute infectious diseases while neglecting the prevention and control of the others.
2. It had paid close attention to infected areas while neglecting areas less frequented by epidemics.
3. Public participation in epidemic prevention and control fell short of expectation.
4. It had failed to mobilize adequate number of doctors to support epidemic prevention and control in the countryside.
5. Many medical workers still prioritized treatment over prevention.

The Ministry of Health believed that apart from medical measures, it should also emphasize publicity and public education, encourage public participation in disease prevention and control, and engage medical workers in mass activities. Only in this way could every Chinese citizen be made aware of the significance of public health and disease prevention and control. On September 9, 1951, after reading the *Comprehensive Report on Epidemic Prevention in the Past 21 Months* submitted by He Cheng to the CPC Central Committee, Mao Zedong issued an instruction in the name of the CPC Central Committee to all Party committees above the county level. He pointed out: "The Central Committee believes it is a mistake not to attach sufficient importance to sanitation, epidemic prevention, and general healthcare. This mistake must be corrected. In the future, sanitation, epidemic prevention, and general healthcare must be regarded as a major political task that we must attach great importance to." He emphasized that "it is necessary to make public officials realize that, the loss of lives, including both humans and animals, and economic losses caused by lack of health knowledge or lack of access to healthcare may exceed the loss caused by floods, droughts, and other natural disasters. We must attach equal importance to healthcare and disaster relief. We must never neglect healthcare."[4] It was the first document on healthcare personally drafted by Mao Zedong after the founding of the People's Republic of China. This document pointed out the importance of public health and its position in government agenda, preparing the ground for the culmination of the Patriotic Hygiene Campaign led by the CPC and the government.

4 Gao Enxian. 2000. "Documents on Healthcare Approved by Mao Zedong in the Early Days of the Founding of the People's Republic of China." *Journal of Chinese Medical History* 1: 42–45.

2

Since 1952, Chinese citizens from all walks of life have actively participated in the Patriotic Hygiene Campaign launched by the CPC and the Chinese government. On an unprecedented scale, this campaign was not only an effective countermeasure against the germ warfare of the US military but also significantly improved access to sanitation and health in both urban and rural areas of the country and strengthened public hygiene education. The campaign focused on the hygiene of children, bodies, indoor settings, yards, streets, kitchens, toilets, and livestock pens, and the eradication of flies, mosquitoes, lice, fleas, bed bugs, and rats. A slogan said, "Killing a fly is equivalent to defeating an American enemy."[5] All Chinese people, men and women, old and young, united as one and achieved brilliant results. The national campaign culminated in June and it was estimated that more than 14 million people in Shandong Province, Beijing, Tianjin, and Chongqing participated in it. About 50 per cent to 60 per cent of farmers in Jilin Province participated in the campaign regularly. A large number of health workers were trained to facilitate this campaign. For example, Zhejiang Province, Shenyang City, Jinan City, and Changwei City have trained more than 640,000 health workers. Evening schools nationwide also offered sanitation and hygiene training programs to workers and farmers. For example, in Shenyang, Andong, Nanjing, Jinan, and Hangzhou, more than 2 million people participated in sanitation and hygiene training programs.

This campaign significantly improved access to sanitation and health care across the country. On the front of pest control, it was estimated that Zhejiang Province and Beijing, Tianjin, Shenyang, Fushun, Anshan, Benxi, Nanjing, Jinan, Qingdao and other cities killed two and a half tons of flies and more than one ton of larvae. Many areas strengthened garbage, sewage, and water source management and built public toilets. For example, Shandong Province and Hebei Province had cleared more than 1,807,000 tons of waste by mid-June 1952. Residents in the third district of Nanjing removed the trash accumulated since the Taiping Heavenly Kingdom period in the mid-19th century. Shenyang City dredged 748 kilometers of ditches from March to April. Chongqing City had repaired 670 kilometers of ditches by the end of June. Over 135,000 toilets were repaired or built in 27 cities and counties in Songjiang in March and April. Most wells in the rural areas of Jilin, Heilongjiang, and Western Liaoning were equipped with a cover. By the end of May, Tianjin had filled or disinfected

5 Li Dequan. "Public Health in China in the Past Three Years." *Xinhua Monthly*, October 1951, 47.

4,000 *mu* (65.89 acres) of sewage pits. It blocked more than 420,000 rat holes and tree holes.[6] In major cities, sanitation of catering venues, meat stalls, hotels, public baths, and salons was significantly improved under the supervision of health authorities. Many of these venues installed screen windows and doors, covering food to protect it from dust and flies. Many shop assistants put on white uniforms and masks. Some cities also stipulated that catering businesses must disinfect utensils with boiling water before use. Families took hygiene measures to keep their homes and surroundings clean. They also cleaned livestock pens and bathrooms frequently. Regarding personal hygiene, people were advised to take baths, wash clothes and bedding frequently, and not to drink unboiled water or eat cold food. All this shows that the Patriotic Hygiene Campaign not only improved public health but also instilled healthy habits in citizens. On January 23, 1956, the Central Political Bureau of the CPC issued the *National Agricultural Development Program (Draft)*, stating that "starting from 1956, we should strive to eliminate rats, sparrows, flies, and mosquitoes within five, seven or twelve years." Under the call of the CPC Central Committee, the country launched a larger-scale campaign to eliminate the four pests.

Pest control and disposal of garbage and sewage were the most common elements of the Patriotic Hygiene Campaign. Cleaning and pest control activities were carried out regularly and irregularly during spring, summer, and autumn when the incidence of infectious diseases was high, as well as on the Spring Festival, Labor Day, Dragon Boat Festival, National Day, and other holidays. According to data collected, about 90 per cent of urban residents and 60 per cent of rural residents regularly participated in the Patriotic Hygiene Campaign.[7] Led by local governments, people cleaned rivers, ditches, and puddles that had been long polluted before liberation. Longxugou Ditch in Beijing, Wulao Village in Nanjing, Hengbin River in Shanghai, and Jinzhong River, Qiangzi River, Chilong River, and Sifangkeng in Tianjin were all infamous for pollution before liberation. After the founding of the People's Republic of China, especially after 1952, the environment in these places had been greatly improved. For example, Wulao Village in Nanjing was known as a "Distressed Village" in the past. During the Patriotic Hygiene Campaign, the villagers cleared the garbage accumulated for decades, filled polluted ponds, ditches and depressions, constructed new roads, improved public restrooms, and planted trees and flowers. To improve sanitation and hygiene, a dedicated

6 Feng Luren. "Patriotic Hygiene Campaign Achieved Great Results." *Xinhua Monthly*, August 1952, 1.

7 Cui Yitian. 1957. "First Public Health Project in China during 1953–1957." *Medical History and Health Organizations* 4: 246.

organization was established, policies formulated, and public education carried out. As a result, the dirty, smelly village that used to attract lots of mosquitoes was turned a clean and tidy place where villagers lived happily. Due to the active public participation in the Patriotic Hygiene Campaign, flies, mosquitoes, mice, and sparrows in the country decreased significantly. The campaign played an influential role in preventing diseases and improving the environment and citizens' personal hygiene and health.

Thanks to the Patriotic Hygiene Campaign, several deadly infectious diseases in China were controlled. Cholera, which had been around for more than 100 years in the country, was wiped out after the founding of the People's Republic of China in 1949 due to effective preventive measures. Smallpox, an infectious disease that had broken out almost every year before 1949, almost disappeared around 1956 in the country except for a few border areas thanks to widespread vaccination. The plague prevalent in China's Inner Mongolia, Jilin, Fujian, Zhejiang, Jiangxi, Hunan, Guangdong and other provinces for a long time was eradicated a few years after the founding of the People's Republic of China. The incidence of other infectious diseases also dropped significantly. For example, from 1951 to 1956, the incidence of typhus and relapsing fever decreased by 89 per cent and 91 per cent, respectively. Schistosomiasis was endemic in 350 cities and counties in 12 provinces in the Yangtze River Basin, affecting nearly 10 million patients. After the founding of the People's Republic of China, the CPC and the Chinese government began to pay attention to the prevention and treatment of this disease. In 1955, the CPC Central Committee issued important instructions on preventing and treating schistosomiasis. In 1956, the *National Agricultural Development Program (Draft)* set out the goal of eradicating the disease in about seven years. From 1949 to the first quarter of 1957, 760,000 patients with schistosomiasis were treated nationwide, and great progress was made in eradicating Oncomelania hupensis, an intermediate host of the disease. In 1956, Oncomelania hupensis was eradicated across one billion square meters of land area. Many local governments strengthened the prevention and control of schistosomiasis through integrated measures such as fecal management and personal protection. Malaria had also been around in China for a long time. After the founding of the People's Republic of China, the country established 49 specialized prevention and treatment centers (stations) and 72 specialized teams in malaria-endemic provinces and regions. It produced dozens of tons of antimalarial drugs each year which, together with other antimalarial Chinese medicines, were used to treat a large number of patients every year. In 1956, more than 445,000 patients with malaria in Guizhou Province received treatment and nearly 700,000 people took preventive medicine. The incidence rate in Mangshi, Yunnan, known as the City of Malaria in the past, was 70 per cent in 1952 and dropped to 6 per cent in 1956. Simao was also an area seriously affected by malaria. By 1956, the disease in Simao had been brought under control. Although there was a major flood in the country in 1956, the number of patients still fell 70 percent from 1955.[8] More than 1,330 sanitation and disease control stations had been established nationwide by the end of June 1957, an eightfold increase compared with 1952. The campaign has led to better access to health services in China. By the end of June 1957, there were more than 4,800 hospitals and nursing homes nationwide, and the number of hospital and nursing home beds increased to more than 339,000, which was more than double the number of beds in 1952 and more than four times the number of beds in 1947. By June 1957, the number of health and medical organizations such as urban and rural health centers/ stations established by the state had grown to more than 23,400, an increase of more than 0.7 times over 1952 and 52.7 times from the pre-1949 level.[9]

There are three main reasons why the 1952–1956 Patriotic Hygiene Campaign achieved such great results. First, the CPC and the Chinese government attached great importance to the campaign. For example, Jinan's mayor personally oversaw the campaign. Below the city level, heads of districts, townships, villages, factories, and schools also assumed responsibility for overseeing the implementation of the campaign in areas over which their authority extended. A top-down approach was adopted with the heads held responsible for mobilization and targets cascading from the top down to the bottom. The city also convened meetings of public officials, various representatives, activists, citizens, and residents/villagers to pass on instructions from superiors and discuss, formulate and implement specific work plans.

Secondly, people actively participated in this campaign. This large-scale mass campaign fully demonstrated the superiority of people's democracy and the tremendous power exerted by the people under this system. Under the leadership of the CPC, Chinese people realized the importance of the campaign to public health and the development of national strength. They actively participated in it just like they actively participated in the War to Resist the U.S. Aggression and Aid Korea, the suppression of counter-revolutionaries, the Land Reform, the movements against "three evils" and "five evils", and the Agricultural Collectivization Movement.

8 Cui Yitian. 1957. "First Public Health Project in China during 1953–1957." *Medical History and Health Organizations* 4: 249.

9 Unknown author. 1958. "Development of Healthcare in China in the Past Five Years." *Xinhua Bimonthly* 3: 113.

Third, with the efforts of the CPC and the Chinese government, the People's Republic of China made remarkable progress in promoting public health and disease prevention and control, laying a solid foundation for advancing the Patriotic Hygiene Campaign. Of course, there were regional disparities in the implementation of the campaign. The campaign did not cover some rural areas, and failed to complete the targets. Even in areas where the campaign was carried out in full swing, there was still a lot of work to be done.

3

In October 1957, in response to the call of the Third Plenary Session of the Eighth CPC Central Committee, the Chinese government once again launched a Patriotic Hygiene Campaign centered on the eradication of the four pests. Many public officials participated in the promotion of the campaign and the eradication of the four pests. On January 8, 1958, the CPC Central Committee issued a notice to launch a winter Patriotic Hygiene campaign centered on the eradication of the four pests and put forward specific requirements. In early January, Mao Zedong conducted an inspection in Xiaoying Alley in Hangzhou City. This exciting news motivated local citizens to actively participate in eradicating the four pests and pay more attention to hygiene. Within two years, the citizens were determined to transform Hangzhou into a clean and beautiful city without rats, sparrows, flies, mosquitoes, stink bugs, cockroaches, or Oncomelania. This inspection also boosted public participation across the country.

In January 1958, in response to the call of the CPC Central Committee, nine provincial and municipal leaders from Liaoning, Heilongjiang, Shandong, Anhui, Jiangsu, Shanxi, Henan, Fujian, and Beijing delivered their radio addresses for public mobilization, and the number of listeners exceeded one million. Leaders of nine provinces and cities, including Jilin, Anhui, Shandong, Hebei, Zhejiang, Henan, Sichuan, Beijing, and Shanghai, personally presided over the local pep rally. Some provinces and cities convened teleconferences and meetings of cadres, representatives of activists, and role models to mobilize the masses. Many leaders participated in the campaign, solved problems arising in the implementation of the campaign in time, and designed slogans and goals, which significantly boosted the general public's enthusiasm and pushed forward the campaign.

In the frigid winter, many public officials and citizens across the country participated in the eradication of the four pests, pushing the campaign to one climax after another. During the 20 days from January 14 to February 4,

1958, people in Anhui Province killed more than 32.1 million sparrows, more than 49 million rodents, more than 1.2 million pots of flies, more than 200,000 pots of mosquitoes, and more than 1.2 million catties of fly pupae. They removed more than 400 million buckets of garbage. On average, each person in the province caught more than two rats. In Changchun City, Jilin Province, 400,000 people used 354 cars, 1,696 horse-drawn carriages, 3,592 trolleys, and 10,998 sledges to clear the thick snow on 273 roads in 10 days. By January 25, six streets in the city had become rat-free, and 3,028 rat control specialists had been trained. In Li County, Hebei Province, 50,000 CPC and Communist Youth League members and nearly 10,000 citizens participated in the campaign, and 218 corps, 1,054 squads, 2,340 reconnaissance teams, and 156 firearm teams were established by young people. Twenty joint defense departments were set up. These personnel were dispatched to different county areas to eradicate the four pests. From mid-December 1957 to mid-January 1958, Li County eradicated rats and sparrows and killed overwintering mosquitoes and flies in more than 20,000 vegetable cellars and dark rooms. The government of Anguo County divided the county into 170 zones, trying to eradicate rats, sparrows, and overwintering mosquitoes and flies. It used 7,045 traps to eliminate almost all sparrows in the county in only half a month. Before the Spring Festival, the county government once again mobilized citizens to step up pest control, leading to another campaign climax.[10] Henan, Shandong, Beijing, Shanghai and other provinces and cities also established large pest control teams and achieved remarkable results in eradicating the four pests.

On March 20, 1959, *The People's Daily* published an editorial entitled "Greater Victory in Fighting Diseases". It pointed out that "the progress in eradicating pests and diseases in 1958 was remarkable, but we must not be complacent with the achievements. We are still far from achieving the goal of eradicating diseases nationwide. It's a very arduous and complicated task. Regional disparities are in progress, and the work in some areas is not yet satisfactory. Vectors and intermediate hosts of infectious diseases, such as mosquitoes, flies, and Oncomelania, breed very quickly. If they are not eradicated, and if we slacken the control efforts for just a while, they will reproduce very fast. Therefore, we must continue to fight pests and diseases." The editorial also said, "The disease control goal in 1959 was to eradicate rats, sparrows, flies, and mosquitoes, and schistosomiasis, malaria, filariasis, kala-azar, hookworm disease and other endemic diseases that posed most serious threats to human health. This

10 Li Xiuzhen. 1958. "Main Reasons for Unprecedented Climax of the Patriotic Hygiene Campaign Centered on Eliminating of The Four Pests." *Medical History and Health Organizations* 1: 2.

glorious political task is part of this year's bigger, better, and more comprehensive Leap Forward Campaign."

After the Spring Festival in 1959, Beijing, Shanghai, Bengbu, and other cities combined pest control and sanitation with fertilizer production. Many small and medium-sized towns and rural areas encouraged public participation in sanitation and fertilizer production activities. From January to May that year, 13 provinces and cities, including Jiangsu, produced seven billion tons of fertilizer in total. Areas prone to schistosomiasis and malaria increased weeding and Oncomelania control efforts to prevent schistosomiasis and adopted effective measures to prevent the relapse of malaria. By the end of May, areas, where Oncomelania control activities had been carried out reached more than 300 million square meters, and more than 5 million people had received treatment to prevent relapse of malaria and during crop planting and harvesting days in spring and summer, Hunan, Sichuan, Jiangxi, and other provinces sent a large number of urban medical workers to rural areas. These medical workers lived and worked with villagers, provided medical services, including disease prevention and control, helped communes and production teams train local workers and cooks, and improved the sanitation practices of canteens. This improved public health increased the attendance rate of workers and inspired enthusiasm in workers and farmers. Many areas also increased schistosomiasis control efforts. According to data from thirteen southern provinces and cities, more than 230,000 patients with schistosomiasis, more than 9 million patients with hookworm disease, and more than 1.57 million patients with filariasis in these provinces and cities were cured.[11][9] Other infectious diseases (such as malaria), venereal diseases, and endemic diseases (such as goitre and Kashin-Beck disease) were also eradicated or controlled in many endemic areas.

Disease eradication is a common dream of human beings. It is a challenging task and requires a lot of efforts in the long run. After founding the People's Republic of China, the CPC and the Chinese government led the masses in multiple Patriotic Hygiene campaigns, eradicating some of the most prevalent diseases that posed a severe threat to public health and significantly improving the health of Chinese people. The fundamental purpose of these campaigns was to eradicate diseases, improve the health of citizens, ensure the smooth progress of the socialist revolution and construction, instill good habits in citizens, and promote sanitation and hygiene practices.

---

11 "We Must Strengthen Disease Prevention and Control in Summer and Autumn." *The People's Daily*, July 25, 1959.

Through these campaigns, the CPC and the government accumulated extensive experience. They summarized effective working methods in public health, which were further improved in the Patriotic Hygiene Campaign from October 1957 to 1959. In summary, under the leadership of the CPC, the Chinese government adopted a proactive approach and comprehensive prevention and control measures, integrated disease prevention and control into development, combined science and technology with mass movements. It made a continuous effort to fight diseases.

CHAPTER 10

The "Eradicating Four Pests" Campaign of the People's Republic of China

Zhao Sheng and Su Zhiliang *

Abstract

The Eradicating Four Pests Campaign was first mentioned in the *17-Point Agriculture Policy*, and the original purposes of the campaign were to improve public health and to increase the country's grain output. Mao Zedong, who attached great importance to the campaign, personally led its publicity and revision of its programmatic document and included it in the *60-Point Working Methods*. With the central government's support, the campaign peaked in the winter of 1957 and the first half of 1958. While it positively reduced the populations of mosquitoes, flies, rats and other vectors, prevented and controlled the spread of infectious diseases, and improved public health, the campaign did increase food production. Impetuously designed and overambitious just like many other campaigns at the time, it harmed to the harmony between man and nature.

Keywords

the Eradicating Four Pests Campaign – Mao Zedong – Great Leap Forward

Many studies have examined the Eradicating Four Pests Campaign as an important part of the broader Patriotic Hygiene Campaign.[1] However, the

---

* Zhao Sheng, Ph.D. in history, associate researcher at the Institute of Contemporary Anhui Studies, Anhui Academy of Social Sciences; Su Zhiliang, professor at the School of Humanities, Shanghai Normal University.

1 Such studies include *Health Care in Contemporary China*, published by China Social Science Press in 1986, *History of Health Care in China* written by Chen Haifeng and published by Shanghai Science and Technology Press in 1993, *A Study of the Patriotic Hygiene Campaign (1949–1959)* by Xiao Aishu, published in the first issue of *Contemporary China History Studies* in 2003, *Mao Zedong and the Patriotic Hygiene Campaign* by Xiao Aishu, published in the fourth issue of *Qinghai Social Sciences* in 2003, and A Review of Studies on the Patriotic

 | DOI:10.1163/9789004737990_011

original purposes and features of the Eradicating Four Pests Campaign and the relationship between Mao Zedong and the campaign have seldom been discussed. To fill these gaps, this study explores the ins and outs of this movement.

1 Launching the Eradicating Four Pests Campaign

In mid-November 1955, Mao Zedong convened in Hangzhou and Tianjin meetings of Party secretaries of 15 provinces, municipalities and autonomous regions in the country's eastern, central south, northeastern, and northern parts. Participants discussed the prospect of agricultural cooperatives and the development of agriculture. After the meetings, Mao formulated the *17-Point Agriculture Policy*, which contained the summary of the discussions and some of his personal opinions,[2] and the Eradicating Four Pests Campaign was introduced in Section 13 of this document. "We should rid the country of the four pests, *i.e.*, rats (and other animals that bring harm to human beings), sparrows (and other birds that bring harm to human beings but further research is required to decide whether we should eradicate crows), flies, and mosquitoes within seven years."[3] The concept of the "four pests" was mentioned for the first time in this document. On December 21, Mao Zedong personally drafted the *Request for Comments on the 17-Point Agriculture Policy*, asking the Shanghai Bureau and CPC committees of provinces and autonomous regions to "convene meetings of local CPC committee secretaries, including some county-level CPC committee secretaries, to conduct in-depth research on the relevant matters."[4] On January 12, 1956, an article entitled "Fighting the Four Pests" was published on the front page of *The People's Daily*, calling for "a nationwide mass campaign to eliminate the four pests within the next seven years (i.e., by 1962)." This was Peoples Daily's first detailed discussion of the Eradicating Four Pests Campaign. On January 25, after a discussion at a highest-level state affairs conference, the Chinese government issued the *National Programme for Agricultural Development (1956–1967) (Draft)* (hereinafter referred to as the "Program"). An expansion of the *17-Point Agriculture Policy,* the Program

Hygiene Campaign in Recent Years written by Li Zidian, published in the third issue of *Beijing CPC History Studies* in 2010.

2 Bo Yibo. 2008. *Review of Several Major Decisions and Events*. History of Chinese Communist Party Publishing House, 368–369.

3 CPC Central Literary Research Department. 1991. *Manuscripts by Mao Zedong after the Founding of the People's Republic (Volume 5)*. Central Party Literature Press. 481.

4 CPC Central Literary Research Department. 1991. *Manuscripts by Mao Zedong after the Founding of the People's Republic (Volume 5)*. Central Party Literature Press. 482.

contained 40 sections, and Section 27 set out the goal of the Eradicating Four Pests Campaign: “Starting from 1956, we should work to eradicate rats, sparrows, flies, and mosquitoes in all areas possible across the country within five, seven or twelve years.”[5] Here, the specified time frame for eradicating the four pests, seven years in the *17-Point Agriculture Policy*, was changed to “five, seven or twelve years”, and the modifier “in all areas possible” was added. Mao Zedong deemed the revision appropriate because of “the addition of the modifier”.[6]

Before this 12-year agriculture development plan was formulated, the Eradicating Four Pests Campaign had already been included in the *17-Point Agriculture Policy*. The article published in *The People's Daily* elaborated on the original purpose of the campaign: “The elimination of rats, mosquitoes, and flies can effectively stop the spread of some acute infectious diseases, reduce the threats from these diseases, and therefore protect the health of citizens. It is essentially a public health initiative.” The article further pointed out that “the primary purpose of the agriculture sector is to increase grain production. The state has taken a series of measures to increase grain output, and farmers have worked very hard in the fields. However, rats, sparrows, and other pests have greatly reduced grain output and caused significant damage to grain storage. Therefore, eliminating rats, sparrows, and other pests is a fundamental way to reduce grain loss and increase the output of grain and cash crops.” To demonstrate the necessity of eliminating rats and sparrows, the article went to great lengths to estimate grain loss caused by rats and sparrows in the country. “Each rat eats about eight *qian* (a traditional Chinese unit of weight) of grain per day, that is, about 18 catties of grain per year. According to a report by the Ministry of Grain, almost all the national granaries have rat nests, and rats store grain in their nests. It is estimated that more than 350 million catties of grain are stolen by rats yearly.” “In 1953, on average, in Kangbao County of Hebei Province, one *dou* (16 catties) of grain was dug out of each rat nest. The country's arable land was 150,000 hectares. Provided that there were six rat nests per hectare of arable land, rats caused more than 14 million catties of grain loss to the county annually.” “According to experiments conducted by the Institute of Zoology of the Chinese Academy of Sciences, a sparrow weighing 19 grams eats five and a half grams of millet a day, about three liters a year. Although it is impossible to count the number of sparrows in the country, it can be estimated that grain

5 CPC Central Literary Research Department. 1994. *Collection of Major Government Documents of the People's Republic of China (Volume 8)*. Central Party Literature Press. 56.

6 CPC Central Literary Research Department. 1992. *Manuscripts by Mao Zedong after the Founding of the People's Republic (Volume 6)*. Central Party Literature Press. 17.

loss caused by sparrows is no less than that caused by rats."[7] A primary purpose of the *National Programme for Agricultural Development* was to "rapidly and significantly increase agricultural production by promoting agricultural cooperatives, and to develop farming, forestry, animal husbandry, fishery, and other agricultural activities."[8] The programme set out the following goal: "Starting from 1956, within 12 years, the average annual grain output in areas north of the Yellow River, the Qinling Mountains, and the Bailong River will increase from more than 150 catties in 1955 to 400 catties; that in the areas south of the Yellow River and north of the Huaihe River will increase from 208 catties in 1955 to 500 catties; that in areas south of the Huai River, the Qinling Mountains, and the Bailong River will increase from 400 catties in 1955 to 800 catties."[9] The original purposes of the Eradicating Four Pests Campaign, which was an essential part of the Program, were to improve public health and to increase the country's grain output.

2 Mao Zedong and the Eradicating Four Pests Campaign

After the programme was promulgated, the central and local government departments competed to complete their tasks ahead of schedule.[10] "After the promulgation of the *National Programme for Agricultural Development*, which contains forty articles, in order not to be labelled as Right conservative, the relevant departments scrambled to make plans, requesting their subordinate units to achieve overambitious targets within short time limits." "The goals set out in the *National Programme for Agricultural Development* were to be completed in five, seven, or twelve years, but some officials were hasty and tried to

7 "Eradicating the Four Pests." *The People's Daily*, January 12, 1956.

8 CPC Central Literary Research Department. 1994. *Collection of Major Government Documents of the People's Republic of China (Volume 8)*. Central Party Literature Press. 69.

9 CPC Central Literary Research Department. 1994. *Collection of Major Government Documents of the People's Republic of China (Volume 8)*. Central Party Literature Press. 49.

10 As early as October 1955 at the Sixth Plenary Session of the Seventh CPC Central Committee, Mao Zedong published the Report on Issues Relating to Agricultural Cooperatives, criticizing right-wing thinking in the socialist transformation of agriculture. This conference greatly drove socialist transformation in handicraft and private industry and commerce to a climax. "Just as the key to driving socialist transformation to a climax is agriculture, he (Mao Zedong) also believed agriculture was the key to speeding up economic growth." (See Bo Yibo. 2008. *Review of Several Major Decisions and Events*. History of Chinese Communist Party Publishing House. 245, 368.) The Program was formed at a time when right-wing thinking was lambasted.

complete all these goals within two or three years."[11] The Ministry of Health quickly formulated the *Plan for the Elimination of the Four Pests and Diseases*, setting out the following goals: "In 1957, cities and industrial and mining areas should be basically free of rats. Rural areas should first encourage villages to eradicate rats. Within four years, all villages and areas within a ten-kilometer radius of the villages should be rats-free. Pastoral areas should eradicate rats within seven years. Before the end of 1956, there should be no sparrows within cities and villages and areas within a one-kilometre radius of cities and villages; within two years, there should be basically no sparrows within a three – or four-kilometre radius of cities and villages; the country should basically eradicate sparrows within three to four years."[12] The aggressive approach to agricultural development spread to other sectors of the economy, and many industries in the secondary sector also set unrealistic targets.

This impetuous tendency caught Zhou Enlai's attention. At the two meetings at the end of January, he said, "We should not proceed rashly but make practical plans based on facts." "We should work hard to achieve attainable and realistic goals and avoid right-wring conservatism. We should also avoid chasing impossible or unrealistic goals. Let's not make the mistake of rash advances." To this end, he asked the State Planning Commission and the Ministry of Finance to modify unreasonable goals.[13] Under the leadership of Zhou Enlai, a campaign against rash advances was launched in the economic sector. On June 20, an editorial published in *The People's Daily*, entitled "Opposing Conservatism and Impetuous Tendency", pointed out: "Many comrades only see one side of issues ... When implementing the Program, they failed to prioritize important tasks. They set unrealistic goals and focused too much on what's wanted rather than what's possible, trying to get a million things done at once. They go from one extreme to the other. Mistakes are inevitable." "Of course, all relevant departments at all levels should implement the Program, but how to implement it depends on local realities, and there is no need to insist on uniformity." During the period when people combated rash advances, the Eradicating Four Pests Campaign was not carried out on a large scale.

At the Third Plenary Session of the Eighth CPC Central Committee in September and October 1957, Mao Zedong said: "We had seen a high tide in 1955, but suffered in the following year as a right-wing conservativism and

11 "Opposing Conservatism and Headlong Haste." *The People's Daily*, June 20, 1956.

12 "The Ministry of Health formulates a plan to eradicate four pests and diseases." *The People's Daily*. February 19, 1956.

13 Bo Yibo. 2008. *Review of Several Major Decisions and Events*. History of Chinese Communist Party Publishing House. 374–375.

an effortlessness mood occurred. Three things were swept away: the principle of doing things with greater, faster, better and more economical results; the *National Programme for Agricultural Development*; and the committees for promoting progress.[14] "This meeting was not only the prelude to the Party-wide criticism of the combat against rash advance but also to the agricultural Great Leap Forward. At the meeting, the CPC Central Committee adopted the *Amendment to the National Programme for Agricultural Development (1956–1967) (Draft)*, which essentially mapped out a course of action for the agricultural Great Leap Forward.[15] The programme was "warmly welcomed by people all over the country and motivated farmers to work harder."[16] The Amendment also changed the wording for eliminating the four pests: "From 1956, we should eliminate rats, sparrows, flies and mosquitoes as far as possible across the country within twelve years. The purpose of eliminating sparrows is to protect crops. Sparrows in cities and forest areas may not be eliminated."[17]

Mao Zedong attached great importance to the Eradicating Four Pests Campaign and personally led its publicity activities. On December 4, 1957, *Anhui Daily* published an editorial entitled "We Must Continue the Campaign Until the Four Pests Are Eradicated", pointing out: "Improving hygiene and eliminating the four pests is an arduous, long-term task. We need to change some customs and habits. We must be persistent. But now some people have a Right deviationist idea about the Eradicating Four Pests Campaign. They are not motivated enough because they lack awareness of the harm of the four pests and the importance of eliminating them. They are being irresponsible for national construction and people's health. We must quickly and thoroughly overcome this thinking, make up our minds, and pull out all the stops to eradicate the four pests, driving the campaign to an even greater climax than the one in 1956." "The goals relating to eliminating the four pests proposed in the *National Programme for Agricultural Development* are correct and necessary, and as long as we are willing to work hard, it is possible to achieve the goals ahead of schedule." After reading this article, Mao Zedong wrote to Hu Qiaomu, "This article is good. It

14 Bo Yibo. 2008. *Review of Several Major Decisions and Events*. History of Chinese Communist Party Publishing House. 447.

15 Bo Yibo. 2008. *Review of Several Major Decisions and Events*. History of Chinese Communist Party Publishing House. 478.

16 "Mobilize the masses to discuss the Agriculture Development Program and increase agricultural output." *The People's Daily*. November 13, 1957.

17 CPC Central Literary Research Department. 1994. *Collection of Major Government Documents of the People's Republic of China (Volume 10)*. Central Party Literature Press. 651.

should be publicised via newspaper and radio."[18] The next day, *The People's Daily* reprinted the editorial. On December 27, *Zhejiang Daily* published a report on Wuxing and Nanxun, two fly-free towns thanks to the hard work of every citizen throughout the year, a feature entitled "Wang Ajin Actively Participates in the Eradicating Four Pests Campaign", an editorial entitled "Eradicating the Four Pests" and nine photos related to the campaign. They caught Mao Zedong's attention. On the same day, Mao said to Hu Qiaomu, "Here is a report, a feature, an editorial and a few photos. You can take a look. *The People's Daily* can republish them." On December 30, *The People's Daily* republished these articles and one of the photos. In addition to paying attention to publicity materials, he also asked Xinhua News Agency to report on the Four Pests Elimination and the Patriotic Hygiene Campaigns.[19] With the support of Mao Zedong, state-run newspapers and magazines at all levels went to great lengths to cover the Eradicating Four Pests Campaign. Take *The People's Daily,* for example. It published many major editorials on the campaign during this period, including "Carrying out the Patriotic Hygiene Campaign in Winter" (December 23), "Thanks to the Hard Work of Every Citizen Throughout The Year, Wuxing and Nanxun Have Become Fly-Free Towns" (December 30), "People Across the Country Are Mobilized to Participate in the National Patriotic Hygiene Campaign" (January 24, 1958), and "Mobilizing People Across the Country to Eradicate the Four Pests and Participate in the Patriotic Hygiene Campaign" (February 5, 1958). Beijing was considered an exemplar in implementing the Eradicating Four Pests Campaign among large and medium-sized cities and received extensive coverage from *The People's Daily*.[20]

Mao Zedong personally supervised the revision of the programmatic document for the Eradicating Four Pests Campaign. On December 7, 1957, he noted, "The Central Committee and State Council should issue a joint

18 CPC Central Literary Research Department. 1992. *Manuscripts by Mao Zedong after the Founding of the People's Republic* (*Volume 6*). Central Party Literature Press. 666.

19 CPC Central Literary Research Department. 1992. *Manuscripts by Mao Zedong after the Founding of the People's Republic* (*Volume 6*). Central Party Literature Press. 667–669.

20 Important articles published by *The People's Daily* on Beijing's role in the campaign include *Engaging leaders at all levels in the preparation for the Eradicating Four Pests Campaign and the Health Campaign in Beijing in Winter* (December 4), *Mobilizing citizens to participate in the Eradicating Four Pests Campaign and the Health Campaign in Beijing* (December 13), *The Blitz Week of the Eradicating Four Pests Campaign and the Health Campaign in Beijing has started and Premier Zhou asked government officials to normalize good hygiene practices* (December 23), *Beijing has launched the Eradicating Four Pests Campaign and will focus on the elimination of rats after the New Year* (December 31), *Beijing has launched a four pests eradication competition. Five units have ridden themselves of the four pests and more than 900 units determine to catch up with them as quickly as possible* (January 16, 1958), and *Criteria for the Participation in the Four Pests Elimination and Hygiene Competition in Beijing* (January 20, 1958).

directive, mobilizing the whole country to pay attention to hygiene and to eliminate the four pests ... The People's Daily should follow that with a good editorial." On December 25, he reviewed the draft of the directive and noted that "it still had some problems, more rhetoric than substance, and did not look closely at the rich experience that had already been gained around the country." So he told Hu Qiaomu that revisions should be made in a way that "would make people feel we can fix the problems, boost their confidence, motivate them to take prompt action. The document should clearly explain why the country should come together to protect its people, livestock and crops from the scourge of diseases. This is at the theoretical level. Then it should discuss specific tactics, which should be sensible, feasible, and credible, informed by genuine expertise." "The document should end with Party secretaries' tasks, and such things as newspapers, magazines, radio broadcasts, and regular cleaning and inspection."[21] On February 12, 1958, the CPC Central Committee and the State Council jointly issued the *Instruction on Eliminating the Four Pests and Paying Attention to Hygiene*, noting "the National Patriotic Hygiene Campaign centered on the elimination of the four pests has reached a climax. In all provinces and cities across the country, people are taking an action to eliminate rats, sparrows, flies, and mosquitoes, promote hygiene, and eradicate the most severe diseases that endanger local people. They have also made plans to meet the goals in the *Amendment to the National Programme for Agricultural Development* (*Draft*) ahead of schedule."[22] On February 13, *The People's Daily* published an editorial entitled "We Must Eradicate the Four Pests in China", setting the goal of making China a strong and prosperous country without the four pests.

Mao Zedong attached great importance to the Eradicating Four Pests Campaign. He included the elimination of the four pests in the *Sixty-Point Working Methods* (*Draft*). Of the 60 Points, 14 were based on the revised Programme. Mao Zedong said: "Party committees at all levels should focus on agriculture in the socialist country." "These are the fourteen essential points from the *Programme for Agricultural Development*. The forty-article Programme must be fully implemented. The fourteen points are what we should focus on. Once the key link is grasped, everything else falls into place."[23] Eliminating the four pests was included in the fourteen points. Obviously,

21 CPC Central Literary Research Department. 1992. *Manuscripts by Mao Zedong after the Founding of the People's Republic* (*Volume 6*). Central Party Literature Press. 666–667.

22 "Instructions of the CPC Central Committee and the State Council on Eliminating the Four Pests and Paying Attention to Hygiene." *The People's Daily*, February 13, 1958.

23 CPC Central Literary Research Department. 1992. *Manuscripts by Mao Zedong after the Founding of the People's Republic* (*Volume 7*). Central Party Literature Press. 46–47.

Mao considered the Eradicating Four Pests Campaign to be one of the most essential tasks of the Programme.

Following the central government's call, the national Eradicating Four Pests Campaign quickly peaked after the winter of 1957 began. "Since the beginning of winter, from cities to the countryside, from plains to mountainous areas, tens of millions of people have joined the Patriotic Hygiene Campaign centered on eliminating the four pests, and have achieved brilliant victories. Countless towns, townships, communes, sub-districts and units have worked to eradicate the four pests. The campaign has reached its peak in many areas."[24] During the period, overzealous people did everything with such haste. The Eradicating Four Pests Campaign achieved excellent results. "The Patriotic Hygiene Campaign centered on the elimination of the four pests was launched rapidly throughout the country and achieved great results." As of February 19, according to data from 25 provinces, municipalities and autonomous regions, "more than 300 million rats and sparrows, and more than 246,000 catties (4.54 million boxes) of mosquitoes and flies had been eliminated. More than 3,392,000 catties of fly larvae had been killed. Tens of millions of tons of garbage had been removed. The sanitary condition in urban and rural areas had been greatly improved."[25]

The National Eradicating Four Pests Campaign culminated from the winter of 1957 to the first half of 1958. After that, due to the rapid development of the Great Leap Forward in all sectors of the economy, all departments and agencies were busy completing the production targets, and the scale of the Eradicating Four Pests Campaign began to decline. On March 16, 1960, Mao Zedong wrote in the CPC Central Committee's Instruction on Sanitation, "Our attention to sanitation has somewhat slackened in the past two years because of the Great Leap Forward in production. Now, we should immediately make arrangement, summarise experience, and organize inspections, competitions, and evaluations. The central government is calling on comrades to pay attention to this issue, to restart the Patriotic Hygiene Campaign in which there was a slackening in the past two years, and to achieve remarkable results in 1960, 1961 and 1962." "All citizens, including the young and the old, teachers and students, men and women, should try their best to use fly swatters and other tools to kill as many of the four pests as possible." At the same time, he emphasised: "Stop killing sparrows. We must eliminate bed bugs now. The new slogan is 'Kill rats,

24 "Mobilizing people across the country to eradicate the four pests and participate in the Patriotic Hygiene Campaign." *The People's Daily*, February 5, 1958.

25 "The Eradicating Four Pests Campaign is advancing rapidly, tens of thousands of units have successfully eradicated the four pests, and areas lagging behind are catching up." *The People's Daily*, February 19, 1958.

bed bugs, flies, and mosquitoes'."[26] On April 10, at the Second Session of the Second National People's Congress, the Chinese government passed the Resolution on Achieving the Goals of the National Programme for Agricultural Development in Advance. The Amendment to the National Programme for Agricultural Development (Draft) in 1967 only made one change: the sparrows in the four pests were changed to bed bugs. "Starting from 1956, we should strive to basically eliminate rats, bed bugs, flies, and mosquitoes as far as possible across the country within twelve years."[27] Tan Zhenlin explained this revision in his report: "The sparrows have been eradicated. The grain production has increased yearly, and the damage of sparrows to grain production has been greatly reduced. At the same time, the forest area has significantly increased. Sparrows are natural enemies of insect pests on trees. So, we should stop killing sparrows. Sparrows in the four pests specified in the Programme should be changed to bed bugs."[28]

In the early 1960s, some large and medium-sized cities launched a campaign against the four pests. For example, in Shanghai, "more than one million workers, shop assistants, residents, soldiers, government officials, and suburban farmers actively responded to the call of the Shanghai Municipal Committee of the CPC, setting off a new upsurge in the Patriotic Hygiene Campaign in the spring"; "In Tianjin, a large number of residents responded enthusiastically to the call of the Party to set off an upsurge in the Eradicating Four Pests Campaign and the Health Campaign"; in Hangzhou, "in the past month, countless government officials, PLA officers and soldiers, teachers and students from universities and high schools, and residents participated in the Health Campaign, and all fly and mosquito breeding sites such as rivers, ponds, depressions, manholes, and livestock pens were fully controlled";[29] in Beijing, "the Mass Patriotic Hygiene Campaign centered on improving sanitation and environment, reducing fly and mosquito breeding sites, and strengthening disease

26 CPC Central Literary Research Department. 1996. *Manuscripts by Mao Zedong after the Founding of the People's Republic* (*Volume 9*). Central Party Literature Press. 80–81.

27 "Resolution of the Second National People's Congress of the People's Republic of China on Achieving the Goals of the *National Programme for Agricultural Development* Ahead of Schedule Adopted at the Second Session of the Second National People's Congress on April 10, 1960." *The People's Daily*, April 11, 1960.

28 Tan Zhenlin. "Strive to Achieve the Goals of the *National Programme for Agricultural Development* Ahead of Schedule – Report at the Second Session of the Second National People's Congress on April 6, 1960." *The People's Daily*, April 7, 1960.

29 "The Patriotic Hygiene Campaign, of which the Eradicating Four Pests Campaign is part, is in Full Swing in Shanghai, Tianjin, Jinan, and Hangzhou." *The People's Daily*, March 28, 1960.

prevention and control is in full swing."[30] However, by the early 1960s, China's economy had collapsed. Take agricultural output in rural areas for example. "In 1960, the actual output of grain stood at 287 billion catties, a decrease of more than 26 percent from 390.1 billion catties in 1957; the actual output of cotton was 21.26 million *dan* (one *dan* is equal to 50 kilogram), which was more than 35 percent less than the 32.8 million *dan* in 1957; the actual output of oil crops was 34.05 million *dan*, which was less than one half of the 75.42 million *dan* in 1957; the year-end number of pigs on agricultural holdings stood at 82.27 million, decreased by 56 percent from 145.9 million in 1957; the number of large farm animals on agricultural holdings at the end of the year was 73.36 million, a decrease of 12.5 percent from 83.82 million in 1957. The output of these agricultural products mostly dropped to the levels in 1951, and the output of oil crops was only half of that in 1951."[31] In 1961, comprehensive economic adjustment began according to the principles of "adjustment, consolidation, enrichment and improvement". After 1961, the Eradicating Four Pests Campaign was carried out intermittently.

3 Features of the Eradicating Four Pests Campaign

The Eradicating Four Pests Campaign captured the zeitgeist of that era, the main manifestatiich included the continuous revisions of the timetable, the involvement of Party secretaries, the focus on campaign tactics, and the use of diversified methods of publicity and mobilisation.

Continuous revision of the timetable. At the time, the country was advancing the Great Leap Forward. Many local authorities proposed unrealistic timetables for eliminating the four pests. "Beijing decided to eradicate the four pests within two years, Henan three years, Shanghai three to five years, Jiangsu four years, Shandong, Shanxi, Zhejiang, Fujian, Guangdong, Yunnan, Gansu, Liaoning, and Heilongjiang five years, and Anhui five to eight years. The cities and counties that decided to eradicate the four pests within one year (1958) include Nanjing, Changzhou, Zhenjiang, and Nantong in Jiangsu Province, Jinan, Yangxin, and Shanxian in Shandong Province, Zhengzhou, Kaifeng, Luoyang, Jiaozuo, and Dengfeng in Henan Province, Lanzhou in

30 "Citizens in Shanghai and Beijing are mobilized to eradicate rats, bedbugs, flies, and mosquitoes as a way to celebrate International Workers' Day." *The People's Daily*, March 26, 1960.

31 Bo Yibo. 2008. *Review of Several Major Decisions and Events*. History of Chinese Communist Party Publishing House. 620–621.

Gansu Province, Tunliu in Shanxi Province, and Lixian and Hejian in Hebei Province."[32] In many places, the timetable was revised frequently and the time limit set to achieve the goal was repeatedly shortened. For example, at the Four Pests Elimination Competition Conference in Beijing, "local authorities challenged each other to eradicate the four pests following higher requirements within a shorter time frame."[33] In Shanghai, "while some units had previously planned to eradicate the four pests within ten or eight years, responding to the demand of the people, they have now revised their plans and shortened the time limit to two years, three years, one year or even just a few months."[34] Jieshou County of Anhui Province, eliminating the four pests, revised its plan three times, changing the time limit from five years to two years, then to one year, and even to merely five months."[35]

Involvement of Party secretaries. The CPC Central Committee and the State Council pointed out in the Instructions on Eliminating the Four Pests and Paying Attention to Hygiene: "The first secretaries of Party organizations in all localities must personally lead this campaign, overseeing planning, publicity, inspection, and evaluation. They need to see to it the heads of subordinate units assume their due responsibility."[36] Therefore, Party and government leaders at all levels in provinces, municipalities, and autonomous regions across the country attached great importance to the campaign, and many senior CPC leaders personally oversaw the implementation of the campaign. "The Shanghai Party and government leaders changed their mobilization method. In the past, mobilization meetings had to be held at various levels to get work done. Now the senior leaders took charge directly and encouraged cadres and the masses to participate in the campaign. This soon brought the campaign to reach its peak. The secretaries of the Jiangsu Provincial CPC Committee and Nanjing Municipal CPC Committee, the mayor of Nanjing City, and many other leaders have worked with the masses to clean roads and kill mosquitoes

32 "Instructions of the CPC Central Committee and the State Council on Eliminating the Four Pests and Paying Attention to Hygiene." *The People's Daily*, February 13, 1958.

33 "Beijing has launched a four pests eradication competition. Five units have ridden themselves of the four pests and more than 900 units determine to catch up with them as quickly as possible." *The People's Daily*, January 16, 1958.

34 "Representative Jin Zhonghua reports on the implementation of the Patriotic Hygiene Campaign centered on the eradication of the four pests in Shanghai, which is carried out to make Shanghai a clean and beautiful city." *The People's Daily*, February 13, 1958.

35 Yang Liu. "Following the Mass Line – Jieshou County's Experience in Eradicating the Four Pests." *The People's Daily*, June 2, 1958.

36 Instructions of the CPC Central Committee and the State Council on Eliminating the Four Pests and Paying Attention to Hygiene. *The People's Daily*, February 13, 1958.

and flies. Party and government leaders in many other provinces and cities also personally led the campaign and conducted inspections promptly, which was why the campaign could last for such a long time."[37] In Jianning County, Fujian Province, "secretaries of CPC committees at county and township levels personally led the Patriotic Hygiene Campaign in parallel with production activities."

The focus on blitz tactics. "In early spring, the four pests become active. In summer and autumn, infectious diseases are rampant. In winter, farmers begin to accumulate fertilizer, repair water projects, improve sanitary conditions, and eliminate overwintering mosquitoes and flies. These are great times to organize activities to eliminate the four pests. Clean-ups were also held during the Spring Festival, Labor Day, and National Day. Random activities were also organized before inspections and evaluation."[38] Although the Instructions on Eliminating the Four Pests and Paying Attention to Hygiene emphasized that random activities should be combined with regular activities, random activities were still the main form of campaign activities.

Use of diversified publicity and mobilization methods. To fully mobilize the masses, the CPC Central Committee instructed: "All resources should be mobilized to carry out lively and powerful publicity activities based on local conditions, requirements and concerns of the people. These publicity activities may be conducted via newspapers, radio broadcasts, slideshows, films, and posters. They may also take such forms as neighborhood promotion, door-to-door visits, exhibitions, mass meetings, and residents' group meetings. Newspapers, periodicals, and radio stations should frequently promote the basic knowledge and best practices relating to the elimination of the four pests, sanitation, and disease prevention, and relevant booklets and pamphlets should be compiled and distributed in large numbers to grassroots organizations. Individuals and collectives playing an exemplary role in eliminating the four pests and improving hygiene practices should be praised and rewarded."[39] These requirements were well implemented in many places. Take Jianning County in Fujian Province and Jieshou County in Anhui Province for example. Jianning County "held over ten large-scale meetings, including those using radio stations, to accelerate action towards the goals of the campaign. Counties,

37 Mobilizing people across the country to eradicate the four pests and participate in the Patriotic Hygiene Campaign. *The People's Daily*, February 5, 1958.

38 "Instructions of the CPC Central Committee and the State Council on Eliminating the Four Pests and Paying Attention to Hygiene." *The People's Daily*, February 13, 1958.

39 "Instructions of the CPC Central Committee and the State Council on Eliminating the Four Pests and Paying Attention to Hygiene." *The People's Daily*, February 13, 1958.

communes and production teams also held meetings and promoted the campaign through folk songs, *kuaiban* (a form of rhythmic comic talk) and jingles. It is estimated that the county organized 155 health promotion activities, 55 on-site observations, 198 slideshows and movies about health, compiled and distributed posters to introduce the eight pests, and created folk songs about the Eradicating Four Pests Campaign. Blackboard news, posters (including big-character posters), local radio stations, slogans, leaflets and other publicity tools were also used to promote the campaign."[40] In Jieshou County, "in the first half month after the launch of the campaign, four radio meetings were held, reaching more than 423,000 people. Forty-nine exhibitions were held, displaying comics and charts that showed crops damaged by sparrows, food stolen by rats, clothes that rats bit, and mosquito-borne diseases, reaching more than 2,500 people. Townships and villages organized demonstrations to promote the campaign. Participants held gongs, drums, flags, banners and tools used to eliminate the four pests. Some carried dead pests. More than 87,500 people participated in such demonstrations. More than 1.12 million cadres, Party members, youth league members, commune members and residents attended education meetings held by communes, product teams, towns and cities. Neighborhood promotional activities were carried out at county fairs, reaching more than 97,000 people. 345 science and health lectures centred on eliminating the four pests were held in various parts of the county, and more than 93,000 people attended these lectures."[41] Thanks to extensive publicity, a large number of role models emerged in the campaign.

The Eradicating Four Pests Campaign received broad support across the country when it reached its peak. In the countryside, "because of extensive publicity, there was a massive campaign against the four pests. More than 200,000 people participated in the campaign. They were divided into rat elimination teams, sparrow elimination teams, fly and mosquito elimination teams, and various blitz teams. More than 480,000 tools were used. These people were found in every corner of the country, on roofs and in houses, fields, woods, and haystacks. Their actions were well-coordinated, quickly dealing the four pests a devastating blow. At the tensest moment, the county's Party, government leaders, and citizens worked around the clock for fifteen days. The participation of the masses, scouts, sharpshooters, and snipers made it impossible for

40 Wen Hua. "Eradicating the Four Pests, Paying Attention to Hygiene, and Improving the Environment of the Mountainous Areas – An Introduction to the Patriotic Hygiene Campaign in Jianning County, Fujian Province." *The People's Daily*, February 24, 1959.

41 Yang Liu. "Following the Mass Line – Jieshou County's Experience in Eradicating the Four Pests." *The People's Daily*, June 2, 1958.

the four pests to survive."[42] In cities, "an army composed of workers, peasants, cadres, students, soldiers and residents was eradicating sparrows day after day. People with tools could be found in every corner of cities. Old ladies and small kids were also making loud noises to frighten away sparrows." "Every morning and from 4:00 p.m. to 7:30 p.m., when sparrows were out of their nests and returning to their nests, citizens would work together to chase them.[43]

The campaign positively reduced the populations of mosquitoes, flies, rats and other vectors, prevented and controlled the spread of infectious diseases, and improved public health. However, for various reasons, the campaign did not increase the country's food production. Impetuously designed and overambitious, just like many other campaigns at the time, it did harm to the harmony between humanity and nature. Studying the Eradicating Four Pests Campaign can offer us some inspiration for the research of the Great Leap Forward.

---

42 Yang Liu. "Following the Mass Line – Jieshou County's Experience in Eradicating the Four Pests." *The People's Daily*, June 2, 1958.

43 "Beijing achieved a great victory in the battle against the four pests, wiping out 400,000 sparrows in three days." *The People's Daily*, April 22, 1958.

CHAPTER 11

The Chinese Pharmaceutical Industry's Ultrasound Promotion Campaign during the Great Leap Forward

Zhang Cheng and Hu Huakai[*]

Abstract

During the Great Leap Forward, China's pharmaceutical industry zealously produced many ultrasound devices and applied them widely in various fields. Still, their efforts failed to deliver the desired results. While we may attribute the failure of a single project to scientific, technological or economic factors, the main reason for the failure of this industry-wide campaign was not false exaggeration but a series of mistakes in technology policies.

Keywords

Great Leap Forward – ultrasound technology – pharmaceutical industry

In[1] 1960, there was a nationwide fanatical push in China to produce and apply ultrasound devices. This resulted in a nationwide campaign which, though as influential as the mass campaign of steel production in 1958, needs to be more researched, only briefly described or reviewed in a few diaries, memoirs, and other literature.[2] People often place this campaign on par with other

* Zhang Cheng, Ph.D. candidate, Department of History of Science and Scientific Archaeology, University of Science and Technology of China, and associate professor, College of Humanities and Social Science, Anhui Medical University. Hu Huakai, professor, Department of History of Science and Scientific Archaeology, University of Science and Technology of China.

1 This study is one of the outcomes of the *Study of the Great Leap Forward from the Perspective of History of Technology* (13YJC770063), a project sponsored by the Humanities and Social Sciences Youth Foundation of the Ministry of Education of China.

2 Only a very few studies have focused on this campaign. *National Obsession with Ultrasound in 1960* by Xue Pangao (3rd issue of *China Scitechnology Think Tank* in 2007) is one of them.

 | DOI:10.1163/9789004737990_012

campaigns during the Great Leap Forward due to their lack of knowledge. It was riddled with false exaggerations as any campaign during the same period. However, when we put it in the history of technology, we can find that the mistakes made by the authorities about technological goals and paths were the main reason for its failure. To demonstrate this point of view and shed light on the real reasons for the failure of this campaign, we will focus on the analysis of ultrasound device manufacturing and application in the pharmaceutical industry, which played a prominent role in this campaign.

1 Application of Ultrasound Technology in the Pharmaceutical Industry: Three Phases during the Great Leap Forward

The application of ultrasound technology in the pharmaceutical industry during the Great Leap Forward, marked by the fanatic Ultrasound Promotion Campaign, can be divided into three phases. The campaign took shape when, due to the rapid development of ultrasound technology worldwide, China began to pay attention to and actively promote this technology. In this context, the pharmaceutical industry started experimenting with this technology and achieved some results. After the campaign began, the pharmaceutical industry was among the earliest to participate in this frenzy. Some pharmaceutical enterprises began manufacturing homemade ultrasound devices in large quantities and unquestioningly expanded their application, claiming all these projects yielded remarkable results. In actuality, only a small number of these projects proved viable, most of which had already worked successfully before the campaign, and no projects developed during the campaign eventually outlast it.

1.1 *A Few Pharmaceutical Enterprises' Trials before the Campaign*

While the import of ultrasound technology and its use in the secondary sector had already started after the Second World War, it is in the late 1950s that China began to attach importance to this technology. In the *Outline of Long-Term Plan for the Development of Science and Technology (1956–1967)* formulated in 1956, "improving electricity and ultrasound technologies and expanding their application" was listed as one of the 57 crucial national scientific and technological tasks.[3] It was in this context that some enterprises in textile, machinery,

3 CPC Central Literary Research Department. 1994. *Collection of Major Government Documents of the People's Republic of China (Volume 9)*. Central Party Literature Press. 488.

chemical and other industries started trying to use ultrasound technology in production.

Beijing Pharmaceutical was one of the earliest to do so.[4] At the end of 1959, the factory tried ultrasound to pulverise benzathine penicillin G and achieved initial success.[5] During the same period, in addition to Beijing Pharmaceutical, Shanghai Second Pharmaceutical Company, the Fourth Pharmaceutical Company, and the General Pharmaceutical Company were also interested in ultrasound technology and were preparing to buy a complete set of equipment.[6] However, China at the time needed more essential technology and capabilities to manufacture the equipment, these enterprises were unable to launch their ultrasound projects before the beginning of the Ultrasound Promotion Campaign.

1.2 *Expanded Industrial Application after the Campaign*

At the beginning of 1960, when the Great Leap Forward was underway, the country launched a mass technological innovation and revolution campaign (from now on referred to as the "Mass Technology Campaign"). During the Mass Technology Campaign, in response to the inadequacy of factory-made ultrasound generators, some enterprises mobilised the masses to produce makeshift ultrasound generators and tried to use them for different purposes. Beijing Pharmaceutical learned how to make ultrasound generators from other enterprises and began to expand their application in its factory. Following ultrasound pulverization, it tried to clean ampoules with makeshift ultrasound generators,[7] of which it found worked effectively.[8] After that, it continued with trials to explore diversified uses of makeshift ultrasound generators, claiming impressive results were achieved. Beijing Pharmaceutical's experience was

4 In the secondary sector, ultrasound technology is mainly used to test and process things. Ultrasound can change the state of matter during processing of materials. This is how ultrasound is mainly used in the pharmaceutical industry.

5 "Technological Revolution Office of the Beijing Municipal Committee of the Communist Party of China. Investigation Report on the Use of Ultrasound." Beijing Archives: 001–017 -00185.

6 The Science and Technology Leadership Group and the Health Committee of the Shanghai Municipal Committee of the Communist Party of China. *Makeshift Ultrasound Generator Promotion Campaign and Relevant Documents of the Shanghai Municipal Committee and the Central Committee of the Communist Party of China*. Shanghai Archives: A52-1-43.

7 An ampoule is a small glass vial used to store injection materials and high-purity chemicals that must be insulated.

8 "Reports and Briefings of Light, Chemical, Textile, Electricity, Printing, and Other Industries on Tests and Application of Ultrasound." Beijing Archives: 001–017-00167.

quickly promoted nationwide. On March 24, 1960, the Ministry of Chemical Industry held a national pharmaceutical conference in Shanghai, and the representative of Beijing Pharmaceutical introduced their experience. Immediately following the conference, Shanghai-based pharmaceutical enterprises launched a mass campaign to manufacture and use makeshift ultrasound generators. In just three days, 1,618 were made, and 44 were put into use.[9] With the support of the municipal government, the mass campaign soon spread across the city. Due to the influence of cities like Shanghai, coupled with the support of the government, an upsurge of interest in these generators emerged across the entire country, resulting in a nationwide campaign.

By May 1960, almost all industries in China had jumped on the bandwagon. Pharmaceutical enterprises all over the country started producing ultrasound generators by themselves and used them in various projects. A typical example was Beijing Pharmaceutical which produced more than 5,000 makeshift ultrasound generators and completed more than 200 tests during the campaign and used them in production and daily life.[10] Zhu Kezhen recorded his visit to Beijing Pharmaceutical in his diary on May 13, 1960. He wrote, "We rode to Beijing Pharmaceutical … to see the factory's ultrasound applications … Ultrasound has been used in the field of chemical production. A row of glass tubes can produce 40kg of vitamin B1 per day. I heard the factory plans to triple the output and cut staff members at the same time. We also looked at various ultrasound generators, and the reeds were similar to those we saw in the electronics factory the day before yesterday. Finally, we saw the devices that used ultrasound to reduce heat. In a room where there were iron-making furnaces, several ultrasound generators were installed, and air was blown into the room to reduce the temperature from about 35°C to more than 20°C. According to them, the air pressure forced the airflow to swirl (in the glassware), and the hot air moved outwards while the cold air stayed in the container. So, the air could also be heated by ultrasound."[6] Pharmaceutical enterprises in other cities also followed suit. Wuhan Pharmaceutical Company made a variety of reed ultrasound generators with reeds, including double-head and triple-head ultrasound generators, and used them for the mixing of Analgin, Sulfadiazine, Synmycin, and other products. Xi'an Pharmaceutical Company manufactured

9 Shanghai Municipal Bureau of Chemical Industry. *Report on the Development of the Ultrasound Promotion Campaign*. Shanghai Archives: B76-1-452-7.

10 "Technological Revolution Office of the Beijing Municipal Committee of the Communist Party of China. Investigation Report on the Use of Ultrasound." Beijing Archives: 001–017 -00185.

many types of ultrasound generators, including the single-layer vortex model, double-layer vortex model, gourd-shaped two-tube model, gourd-shaped three-tube model, various ultrasound generators with reeds, simplified reed model, and the cavity model. Guangdong Pharmaceutical Company used ultrasound generators in production of the intermediates of sulfathiazole, iodine extraction, the intermediates of benzathine penicillin G, odorless synmycin, culture media, and preparations.[11] According to official statistics, in 1960, the pharmaceutical industry used ultrasound in the production of 138 synthetic drugs.[12]

1.3 *Only a Small Number of Ultrasound Applications Outlasting the Campaign*

Although the pharmaceutical industry produced many makeshift ultrasound generators, most of them were abandoned after the campaign, so were most of the ultrasound applications. Take Beijing Pharmaceutical for example. The factory ran more than 200 trials at the height of the campaign in 1960. Still, after the end of the campaign in 1961, only 26 were officially used in production, of which 23 yielded remarkable results.[13] According to a survey conducted by the Beijing Municipal Bureau of Chemical Industry, its seven affiliated factories ran 352 ultrasound application projects during the campaign in 1960, of which 129 projects produced desired outcomes. By the end of 1961, only 34 out of the 129 projects were still used in production.[14] Data show that more than 90 per cent of the ultrasound trial projects run by pharmaceutical enterprises were abandoned after the campaign. Even in the remaining 10 per cent, many had been successfully tested before the campaign. Therefore, the campaign did not bring any beneficial changes to the pharmaceutical industry.

11 Hubei Province Ultrasound Conference. *Application of Ultrasound in the Pharmaceutical Industry*. Hubei Provincial Archives: SZ122-2-190.

12 National Economic Commission & National Science and Technology Commission. *Notice on Promoting Experiments and Applications of Ultrasound Technology and Instructions on Research and Development of New Technologies in 1960 Issued by Hubei Provincial Science and Technology Commission*. Hubei Provincial Archives: SZ122-2-187.

13 "Technological Revolution Office of the Beijing Municipal Committee of the Communist Party of China. Investigation Report on the Use of Ultrasound." Beijing Archives: 001–017 -00185.

14 "Briefing and Investigation Report on the Application of Ultrasound by Relevant Enterprises." Beijing Archives: 001–017-00186.

2 Production and Use of Makeshift Ultrasound Generators in the Pharmaceutical Industry during the Ultrasound Promotion Campaign

What kinds of makeshift ultrasound generators were manufactured by pharmaceutical enterprises in the Ultrasound Promotion Campaign? What projects were these devices used for? What results did these projects achieve? Why was that? Exploring these questions from a technical point of view will not only shed light on why many ultrasound devices and applications were abandoned after the campaign but also help us find the real reason why the campaign failed.

2.1 *Manufacturing of Makeshift Ultrasound Generators during the Campaign*

The models of makeshift ultrasound generators manufactured by pharmaceutical enterprises were mostly the same as those manufactured by other industries, mainly including cavity, reed, and vortex models. Among them, the reed ultrasound generators were the most widely used. The prototype of reed ultrasound generators is the Janovsky-Pohlman ultrasound generator, which was invented and first used for industrial purposes by German physicists Reimar Pohlman and Janovsky in 1948.[15] The basic principle of this device is to generate sound or ultrasound by using a high-speed liquid flow to cause resonance of the reed. At that time, the device's application in emulsification and liquid dispersion had already yielded successful results. In 1951, a British researcher P. Alexander, introduced a simple way to make an ultrasound generator with a single-sided blade as its vibrating reed.[16] This method was widely adopted in the Ultrasound Promotion Campaign. The most popular ultrasound generator with a vibrating reed used during the campaign was made by welding the blade of a stabbing knife to a tube.

Due to lack of the data, the number of makeshift ultrasound generators manufactured by pharmaceutical enterprises during the Ultrasound Promotion Campaign was challenging to estimate. Most of these devices did not work correctly due to the following reasons.

First, some devices had low efficiency because of the absence of necessary adjusters, making resonance difficult. Resonance frequency, a crucial concept

15 W. Janovsky and R. Pohlman. 1948. Schall-und Ultraschallerzeugung in Flüssigkeiten für industrielle Zwecke *Zeitschrift für angewandte Physik* 1: 222.

16 P. Alexander. 1951. "Emulsification with acoustic waves." *Manufacturing chemist and aerosol news* 22 (1): 5–8.

here, is the frequency at which the reed in the ultrasound generator vibrates most efficiently. Take the reed ultrasound generator for example. It works best when it has the frequency at which the reed resonates. Only at this frequency can it work most efficiently. When the fluid pressure is fixed, the reed can only resonate when the distance between the nozzle and the edge of the reed is right. In the Janovsky-Pohlman ultrasound generator, the distance between the reed and the nozzle can be adjusted to ensure the resonance frequency. Makeshift reed ultrasound generators were made by welding the blade of a stab knife to a tube, and the position of the blade was fixed and could not be adjusted to ensure the resonance frequency under a given pressure, so the efficiency was extremely low.

Second, some devices were crudely made. They had severe quality problems, were easily damaged, and had a short service life. At the time, most enterprises used non-standard methods to make ultrasound generators. "Steel, iron, copper, silver, aluminium, plastic, enamel, glass, and ceramic were used instead of special steel to make nozzles",[17] but many of these alternative materials were not suitable at all. For example, the reed and nozzle of a standard reed ultrasound generator are made of special stainless steel, while those of a makeshift one were made of other materials. Some of these materials would be deformed under pressure due to insufficient rigidity. Others could not resist cavitation damage[18] and would rust after a period. These quality problems seriously affected the application of makeshift ultrasound generators. According to the statistics from some enterprises, a makeshift device was expected to be in use for only 7 to 14 days and must be replaced afterwards.[19] Such a short service life offsets its cost advantage.

Last but not least, the manufacturing of most makeshift ultrasound generators needed to follow the necessary standards, process flow, or testing methods. During the campaign, the masses designed ultrasound generators found the required materials and made the devices themselves. The masses determined the devices' shape and materials solely based on their work experience. There was no uniform manufacturing standard or process. More importantly, required testing equipment and mature testing methods were generally lacking then. Take the Beijing Municipal Bureau of Chemical Industry, for example.

---

17 "Report on the Use of New Technologies such as Ultrasound and Pipeline Synthesis, drafted by the Ministry of Industry of the Beijing Municipal Committee of the Communist Party of China and related materials." Beijing Archives: 001–015-00372.

18 High-intensity sound waves can create cavities in the liquid. When the cavities rupture, extremely high pressures are generated. This process is called cavitation.

19 Bureau of Chemical Industry. *Briefing on 'Battles' of the Technological Revolution Campaign*. Beijing Archives: 097–001-00137.

It only had three frequency measuring instruments, and none could work appropriately because of missing parts.[20] Under such conditions, makeshift ultrasound generators were generally used without any test, so their quality was hardly guaranteed.

2.2 *Ultrasound Application Projects during the Campaign*

The number of ultrasound application projects during the campaign can be divided into three categories. The first was projects that had successfully passed the required tests and were used for a long time. The second was projects that were technologically or financially inviable despite positive results in initial tests and were thus shelved after the campaign. The third were projects that involved exaggerated or even falsified results and were thus abandoned after the campaign. For example, a survey conducted at the end of 1961 showed that among the 113 ultrasound application projects of 71 key enterprises in the secondary sector in Beijing, only 25 projects had passed the required tests and were in use for a long time, accounting for 22.1 per cent; 45 had passed required tests but were shelved due to various reasons, accounting for 39.8 per cent; 12 projects had been promoted but the results were unsatisfactory, accounting for 10.6 per cent; 31 projects failed to meet technical standards, pending further tests, accounting for 27.4 per cent.[21] The situation in the chemical industry, which pharmaceutical enterprises were part of, was even worse. According to a survey conducted by the Beijing Municipal Bureau of Chemical Industry at the end of 1961, among 352 ultrasound application projects of its seven factories, only 34 projects yielded good results and were still in use, accounting for 9.65 per cent; 95 projects had yielded good results but were no longer in use due to various reasons, accounting for 26.98 per cent; 18 projects had yielded good results and were being improved, accounting for 5.11 percent; 205 projects failed to pass required tests or yield good results, accounting for 58.23 per cent.[22] Based on the data above, the first category of projects accounted for only 10 to 20 per cent, and the second and third categories accounted for 80 per cent to 90 per cent. Although some makeshift ultrasound generators had no quality problem, they could not work effectively because they were not used

---

20 Bureau of Chemical Industry. *Briefing and Investigation Report on the Application of Ultrasound by Relevant Enterprises*. Beijing Archives: 001–017-00186.

21 "Technological Revolution Office of the Beijing Municipal Committee of the Communist Party of China. Investigation Report on the Use of Ultrasound." Beijing Archives: 001–017 -00185.

22 *Briefing and Investigation Report on the Application of Ultrasound by Relevant Enterprises*. Beijing Archives: 001–017-00186.

in the right projects. Most of the application projects were shelved after the campaign.

We believe that ultrasound application in an industrial production project must meet three criteria:

First, it must be scientific. It must conform to the fundamental scientific principles and, more importantly, be tested through experiments. Only applications that have successfully passed the required tests can be applied.

Secondly, technical problems encountered during the use of ultrasound must be solved. The laboratory's technical conditions differ from those required for large-scale industrial production. Even if a project is successfully tested, technical problems must be solved before it can be promoted and applied in the secondary sector.

Finally, it must be cost-efficient, or there is no alternative to the application. Cost is an essential consideration in industrial applications. Ultrasound technology faces competition from other technologies in this regard. Only when ultrasound technology allows the same task to be completed at a lower cost and higher efficiency can it be applied in an industrial project. All ultrasound projects that continued to be used in the pharmaceutical industry after the Ultrasound Promotion Campaign met these three criteria. Conversely, the projects shelved after the campaign failed to meet at least one of the three criteria.

Next, we will analyse three cases, one for each of the three categories of projects, to illustrate these three criteria further.

Case 1: Application of ultrasound in the production of aspirin. This project was abandoned because it was not scientific. The method adopted by the project was to mix salicylic acid and acetic anhydride in a storage tank, heat it to 70°C through a preheating pipe, and use a gear pump to transport it to the reed ultrasound. Liquid was sprayed from the nozzle under pressure to cause the reed to generate ultrasound. It was said that the reaction in the reactor tank required 3–4 hours, and with ultrasound, the reaction could be completed instantly when the liquid passed through the ultrasonic zone.[23] Through a simple analysis, we can see that the results of this project were falsified. According to a basic knowledge of chemistry, with heating and the catalyst, salicylic acid and acetic anhydride can form acetylsalicylic acid (commonly known as

23 Pipelines and Ultrasound. In Ultrasound Office of the Science and Technology Commission of the Shanghai Municipal Committee of the Communist Party of China (Ed.). *16 Technical Documents for Theoretical Studies of Makeshift Ultrasound Generators*. Shanghai Archives: A52-2-959-44.

aspirin) and acetic acid. When the temperature reaches 70°C if no catalyst is added, the reaction will not occur, even if ultrasound is used; if the catalyst is added, this reaction will occur even if ultrasound is not used. What really happened with the project should be that the reaction occurred in the preheating pipe under the influence of the catalyst, and the liquid containing acetylsalicylic acid was sprayed from the nozzle. Ultrasound only had a mechanical effect like stirring in this process and no catalytic effect on the reaction. Many other projects at the time, such as the application of ultrasound to produce nitrofural, ethylenediamine, and vitamin C, were also not scientific. The test results of these projects were all falsified.

Case 2: Ultrasonic cleaning of ampoules. The scientific principle that ultrasonic cleaning is based on is that the acoustic cavitation effect produced by ultrasound can separate dirt and particles from the wall of a container. This project was shelved not because it was not scientific but mainly for the following reasons: First, the technical problem that prevented it from being used in industrial production was not solved. A pharmaceutical company needed to clean tens of thousands of ampoules every day. The large-scale cleaning task required multiple ultrasonic devices to be used at the same time. Still, when a compressor drove multiple ultrasonic devices at the same time, it was challenging to get their vibrating systems to vibrate at their respective resonance frequencies at the same time if their resonance frequencies were different. This technical problem was not solved at the time. Second, it was not cost-efficient. There was already a mature mechanical method for cleaning ampoules, and the ultrasonic cleaning method was still immature and had no advantage compared with it. So, this project was shelved after a period of use in the early stages of the campaign.

Case 3: Ultrasonic pulverization of benzathine penicillin G. The following are the main reasons why this project was still in use after the campaign: Firstly, it was scientific. Ultrasonic pulverization is based on the scientific principle that ultrasonic cavitation can break up the insoluble solids in a liquid into smaller particles. The project had been tested by Beijing Pharmaceutical and was proven to be feasible. Secondly, the production scale of benzathine penicillin G was small, and the technical problem was easy to solve. Beijing Pharmaceutical initially produced only a few hundred grams of this drug daily, so it did not encounter the technical issues relating to large-scale processing, such as the one faced by ultrasonic cleaning. Last, only ultrasound technology can achieve the particle fineness prescribed by the Pharmacopoeia, and no other technology could replace it. For these reasons, the project was still in use after the campaign.

3 Reasons Why the Ultrasound Promotion Campaign in the Pharmaceutical Industry Failed

The success of an ultrasound application depends on whether it is scientific, technologically feasible, and cost-efficient at the same time. Even if an ultrasound application does yield good results, it may not be widely promoted in the industry. The reasons for the failure of the Ultrasound Promotion Campaign in the pharmaceutical industry include mistakes made by policymakers concerning the manufacturing and application of ultrasound devices, formalism, and false exaggerations.

3.1 *It Was a Mistake to Promote Ultrasound Projects as the Main Technological Development Task in the Industry*

Due to an overzealous promotion of ultrasound processing technologies, the decision makers inaccurately assessed the stages of development, leading to misguided directions in the development of some key production technologies in the industry. This misjudgment had significant consequences, affecting the overall progress and success of the industry.

First of all, there were many different ultrasonic processing technologies. Some were mature and had been used in real life, such as ultrasonic pulverization. Some were in the transitional stage from experiment to real-life application, such as ultrasonic cleaning. Some were still in the experimental stage, such as ultrasonic chemistry. Due to the different development stages of ultrasonic processing technologies, it was unrealistic to promote applications of all ultrasonic processing technologies in a short period of time. The correct approach should be promoting a technology only when it can be considered as mature. During the Ultrasound Promotion Campaign, the decision-makers misjudged the maturity of most ultrasonic processing technologies in pursuit of immediate results and believed that the application of these technologies would immediately yield results. The unrealistic, fanatic promotion of ultrasound applications would certainly lead to failure.

Secondly, each industry has its key technologies. It is only wise to promote ultrasound applications in an industry where ultrasound technology can be used. In many sectors, ultrasound technology cannot play such a role. The key technologies in the pharmaceutical industry are associated with pharmaceutical chemistry. At that time, ultrasonic pulverization and ultrasonic cleaning, which were already mature, only played an auxiliary role in production processes. They did not play a vital role in the pharmaceutical industry, so it was unreasonable to fanatically promote them in the pharmaceutical industry. Although ultrasonic chemistry may have an effect on key technologies in the pharmaceutical industry, it is still in the exploratory stage in both theoretical and practical terms. It is still in the experimental stage and has not achieved broad applicability in the secondary sector. Therefore, it was unrealistic to promote such technology in the field of ultrasonic chemistry, which still needed to be mature. At that time, the reason for fostering ultrasonic research and application in the pharmaceutical industry was because it was believed that ultrasound could facilitate chemical reactions and even bring about revolutionary transformation. This belief was based on falsified test results of ultrasound application projects such as the application of ultrasound in aspirin production. Judgments made based on falsified test results fell out of alignment with reality, and the technological development goal set based on such judgments took time to achieve.

3.2 *The Decision-Makers Selected the Wrong Technological Route, Trying to Mainly Use Mechanical Ultrasonic Devices to Meet the Demand for Ultrasonic Applications*

Furthermore, the technological route selected was impossible to achieve the technological development goal, which was unreasonable. Ultrasonic devices can be divided into two categories: electroacoustic and mechanical. The campaign focused on mass production and application of mechanical ultrasound generators instead of electroacoustic transducers with high power and high conversion efficiency. This choice regarding the technological route is debatable.

On the one hand, there were reasons for choosing such a technological route. At that time, most ultrasonic devices were mainly electroacoustic, and different countries manufactured different ultrasonic devices. Europe and the United States primarily manufactured piezoelectric transducers, while the Soviet Union focused on magnetostrictive transducers. China lacked the necessary technology and resources to manufacture these two types of transducers on a large scale. It took a lot of work for China to manufacture piezoelectric transducers made of piezoelectric single crystals on a large scale because of cost considerations. In the case of piezoelectric transducers made of low-priced piezoelectric ceramics, it was challenging to meet the magnetostrictive power requirement because the manufacturing technology of piezoelectric ceramics in China was still immature at that time. Although magnetostrictive transducers have stable mechanical properties and are suitable for use as high-power ultrasound sources, a large amount of nickel is required to manufacture this kind of transducer, and nickel is a scarce resource in China. So, it is also difficult to manufacture this kind of transducer on a large scale in China. In addition, both piezoelectric and magnetostrictive transducers need to be equipped with electric generators. At that time, electron tubes, which were bulky and expensive, were essential components of most electric generators. The costs of manufacturing and using such electric generators were very high. This is why it was difficult for China to manufacture electroacoustic transducers on a large scale at the time. Mechanical ultrasonic devices such as ultrasonic flutes are simple in structure, stable in performance, and low in manufacturing and use costs. They can be used as sources of power ultrasound in some fields. It was reasonable and necessary for China to manufacture mechanical generators at the time. Although it was difficult to promote the application of scientifically developed ultrasound generators on a large scale, some application projects could achieve success. For example, shortly after the campaign, several pilot projects relating to the application of ultrasound generators carried out by the Ultrasound Lab, Institute of Electronics, Chinese Academy of Sciences and Beijing Guanghua Dyeing and Weaving Factory yielded successful results.

On the other hand, this technological route had apparent flaws. First, excessive reliance on mechanical generators means overdependence on one type of energy, which could easily cause a power supply crunch. Secondly, there was also a contradiction between the relatively narrow application range of mechanical generators and the need for extensive use of ultrasound technology. The flaws of this technological route were exposed during the campaign. For example, Shanghai manufactured more than 1.2 million makeshift ultrasound generators during the campaign, but only 400,000 were actually used. One of the main reasons for this was power supply shortages.[24] In addition, there needed to be more confidence in the role of mechanical generators. People regarded them as omnipotent, believing ultrasound was marvellous and could be used anywhere. This belief was not backed by any experiment. It was the reason why ultrasound generators were misused. In fact, different fields and different purposes require different types of ultrasound generators. The question of whether mechanical generators are suitable for a project needs to be answered through trials. Although before the start of the Ultrasound Promotion Campaign, some research institutes affiliated with the Chinese Academy of Sciences and in the secondary sector also conducted preliminary studies on some types of mechanical generators, proving that these generators were effective for uses such as emulsification, dispersion, and pulverization, the scope of this type of research was limited. The fact that the mechanical

24 Report on Solving Problems Relating to Ultrasonic Power. In Ultrasound Office of the Science and Technology Commission of the Shanghai Municipal Committee of the Communist Party of China, ed. *16 Technical Documents for Theoretical Studies of Makeshift Ultrasound Generators*. Shanghai Archives: A52-2-959-48.

generator can be used in a few processes, such as emulsification, does not mean that it can be universally applied in all processes. Trials must be carried out to determine whether it can be used in other methods. Yet, such trials were not carried out during the Ultrasound Promotion Campaign. Although the campaign advocated scientific experiments, ultrasound generators were, in fact, directly used in production activities without being scientifically tested first. Only when mechanical generators were correctly applied could they achieve the desired results.

3.3 *Formalism and False Exaggerations Were also Important Factors That Contributed to the Failure of the Campaign*

Formalism and false exaggerations also affected the results of the campaign. First of all, some departments and enterprises manufacture and apply ultrasound generators just for the sake of it, ignoring other concerns, such as practical utility. Some enterprises manufactured many makeshift ultrasound generators but needed to put them into use. There were many reasons why they were not used, and formalism was one of the significant reasons. These enterprises were purely pursuing production quantity and never planned to use the products. In some cases, makeshift ultrasound generators were used, but in a meaningless way. In other cases, these generators did not have any practical utility and were installed for show. For example, they were installed near bottle washing nozzles in laboratories, faucets above washbasins, and telephones. These are just some examples of formalism in the campaign. Of course, such an approach could not lead to any results.

Secondly, exaggerated results and false theoretical explanations fueled the fanaticism about ultrasound technology. The applicability of ultrasound was hugely exaggerated in the campaign. Some people said ultrasound was the "panacea", had "magical effects", and could be used everywhere to achieve everything. For example, some enterprises claimed that in case of an abnormal position of the fetus, the fetal position could be corrected by using an ultrasound device to scan the toes of the pregnant woman.[25] Such exaggerations and misinformation contributed to ultrasound technology's zealous promotion and application. Some theorists also jumped on the bandwagon, "inventing" various theories to provide explanations for impossible phenomena. For example, some research departments once proposed the ultrasonic jet theory, trying to systematically explain the effectiveness of makeshift ultrasound

25 Office of the Industrial Products Research Commission of the Shanghai Municipal Committee of the Communist Party of China. *Briefing on the New Technology Conference*. Shanghai Archives: A53-2-160-1.

generators. Some enterprises proposed analyzing the effect of ultrasound on the motions inside matter. They proposed contradictory hypotheses and methods to diagnose technical problems relating to ultrasound. Some even said ultrasound could correct the abnormal position of the fetus and used the traditional meridian theory to explain this. These false theoretical explanations were very misleading at that time.

It should be noted that the failure of the Ultrasound Promotion Campaign in the pharmaceutical industry was primarily attributable to the inappropriate technological goal and route. Although formalism and false exaggerations were severe problems, there were other reasons for the campaign's failure. In other words, the campaign would only succeed with formalism and false exaggeration. Moreover, in many cases, it was precisely because of mistakes made by policymakers that all kinds of unrealistic requirements were put forward, giving rise to all forms of formalism and false exaggerations.

Based on the above analysis, we can draw the following conclusions regarding the Ultrasound Promotion Campaign in the pharmaceutical industry: First, some ultrasound application projects in the sector were shelved because they failed to meet the three requirements at the same time – being scientific, being technologically feasible, and being cost-efficient. This conclusion is also applicable to ultrasound application projects in other industries during that period. Second, the failure of the Ultrasound Promotion Campaign on an industrial scale was attributable primarily to mistakes relating to technological policy and, secondly, to formalism and false exaggeration. To answer the question of whether this conclusion applies to other industries, we will need to analyse the specific circumstances of different sectors. Many issues of the Ultrasound Promotion Campaign, an event in the history of science and technology with extensive social impact during the Great Leap Forward, are worth studying. More in-depth and detailed research is needed to have a more comprehensive understanding of the causes and consequences of the campaign.

CHAPTER 12

On Beijing's Family Planning Campaign in the 1960s

*Wang Linran**

Abstract

In the 1960s, Beijing launched a family planning campaign because of the rapid population growth and other factors that pressured economic and social development. During the campaign, Beijing set up family planning organizations at different levels, identified and trained a team of leading communication specialists, made meticulous communication efforts, and developed a network of contraceptive marketing and medical technologies for birth control. As the first family planning practice, the campaign slowed Beijing's rapid population growth. Although it did not last long, the general public gained a preliminary understanding of family planning, laying the foundation for implementing the family planning policy.

Keywords

1960s – Beijing – family planning – public campaign

The[1] theories and practices concerning the family planning policy have been widely discussed, but the Chinese academic community rarely addresses family planning as part of historical studies.[2] China launched a large-scale urban family planning campaign in the 1960s, marking the beginning of the country's family planning initiative. This paper probes into the family planning campaign in Beijing to seek inspiration.

* Wang Linran, Ph.D. student in the School of History, Beijing Normal University.

1 This paper is an outcome of the research project on "History of Contemporary China" (10&ZD077) supported by the National Social Science Fund of China (NSSFC).

2 The only academic works are Sun Muhan's *History of Family Planning in China* (Northern Women and Children Publishing House, 1987) and Yang Faxiang's "A Study on the History of Family Planning in Contemporary China" (Doctoral Dissertation, School of Humanities, Zhejiang University, 2003). The family planning campaign in the 1960s is addressed in both works, but the issue is not thoroughly analyzed. There is still a shortage of papers on this subject.

 | DOI:10.1163/9789004737990_013

1 The Demographics of Beijing in the Early 1960s

After the founding of the People's Republic of China (PRC), Beijing saw the gradual resumption of production activities, along with greater social stability and improved healthcare facilities, which led to the rapid growth of population. From 1950 to 1963, with the exception of 1961, "the birth rate for Beijing was more than thirty births per thousand people, exceeding forty in five of the years, making the years the first peak period of population reproduction for the capital city".[3] According to a briefing published by the General Office of the CPC Beijing Municipal Committee, the birth rate and rate of natural increase (RNI) for Beijing reached a record high in 1963. "The city's population saw a natural increase of 259,000 people, making the RNI 38.3 per thousand, reaching the highest level in history."[4] If such population growth continued, as relevant authorities held, "the increasing proportion of children in the population of Beijing would worsen the problem of education and cause great difficulties in many sectors such as employment, housing, public transportation, food and supply of commodities".[5] Some districts, counties and organisations conducted surveys on population issues and identified many problems.

Firstly, rapid population growth puts great pressure on economic and social development. The Tuoli People's Commune in Fangshan County produced four hundred thousand kilograms of grain in 1963, hitting a record high, but "still needed ninety-five thousand kilograms of grain rations supplied by the government". After an investigation, Fangshan County found that it was because "grain rations were equally distributed to children and adults, so families with more children would get more rations."[6] In 1949, per capita land ownership in Tixiazhuang production brigade of Henan Village in Miyun County was four *mu* on average, and grain output was eighty-five kilograms per *mu*, so average grain ownership was 387 per capita per year. With the improvement in productivity, the average yield per *mu* reached 130 kilograms in 1963, an increase of fifty-two per cent over 1949. However, because of land occupation by irrigation works and especially the rapid growth of population, the average land area per

3 Editorial Committee of *Beijing Gazetteer*, ed. 2004. *Annals of Beijing: Population*. Beijing: Beijing Publishing House. 246–247.

4 General Office of the People's Committee of Beijing Municipality. "Debriefing (February 5, 1964)." Beijing Municipal Archives: 002–020-00377.

5 Leading Group of Beijing Municipality for Family Planning. "Report on Advancing Family Planning (September 3, 1963)." Beijing Municipal Archives: 002–020-00380.

6 General Office of the People's Committee of Beijing Municipality. "Debriefing (November 26, 1963)." Beijing Municipal Archives: 002–020-00377.

person in that year was two *mu* less than that in 1949, and grain ownership per capita per year was nearly 150 kilograms less than that in 1949.[7]

Secondly, rapid population growth hurts people's lives and work. According to a survey conducted by the Beijing Women's Federation, "seventy to eighty per cent of the frail women and children are from families with more children, the workers in need are also those who have more children, and sixty per cent of the families whose living expenses are less than 12 yuan have more children."[8] Early marriage and early childbearing also affected the development of young people. According to a report by the Beijing Municipal Committee of the Communist Youth League of China (CYLC), some members of the Youth League performed unsatisfactorily at work because they had children. As a result, "most married young people, especially young women, are reluctant to have children early and have more children."[9] According to Ms Wang, a retired teacher now in her seventies, who was assigned to work in a research institute after graduating from university at the beginning of the campaign, "the government encouraged only two children for one family, but I would prefer only one. Many young intellectuals at the time shared the same idea."[10]

Thirdly, some people needed contraception, but their attempts would often fail because of the lack of contraceptives. Before the family planning campaign, people in Tongxian County would use folk prescriptions to prevent pregnancy.[11] The women in the Lugouqiao Commune gave birth to many children, which brought them great pain. They wanted to use contraception, but due to the lack of scientific knowledge they did not know how to do it. Some had to resort to folk prescriptions to prevent pregnancy or have an abortion, which turned out to be ineffective and also did harm to women's health.[12] Obviously, some had the need for birth control, but contraceptives provided by the government were in short supply.

---

7 Office of Beijing Municipal Family Planning Commission. "Family Planning Debriefing (No.10, 1963)." Beijing Municipal Archives: 002–020-00379.

8 Beijing Women's Federation. "Report on Family Planning (October 1963)." Beijing Municipal Archives: 084–002-00295.

9 CYLC Beijing Municipal Committee. "Report on Late Marriage and Family Planning Education to Youths by the Youth League Branch of Fengshan Production Brigade (January 30, 1964)." Beijing Municipal Archives: 100–001-00897.

10 Based on the author's interview with 74-year-old WJ in a university community of Xueyuan South Road, Haidian District, Beijing on August 1, 2013.

11 Beijing Women's Federation. "Family Planning in Suburbs and Related Problems (December 28, 1963)." Beijing Municipal Archives: 084–002-00295.

12 Office of Beijing Municipal Family Planning Commission. "Trial Operation of Medical Teams in Sanluju Production Brigade of Lugouqiao Commune (March 31, 1964)." Beijing Municipal Archives: 002–020-00391.

2 The Organization of Family Planning Campaign in Beijing

If we look at the issue in a broader context, it is easy to find that Beijing's population problem is represented in a microcosm, the one facing the country as a whole at the time. In the first decade of the PRC, birth control was encouraged by some experts or reports, but no concrete measures were taken, and the country's population maintained momentum for rapid growth.[13] In July 1957, economist Ma Yinchu put forward a new theory of population advocating birth control, which was immediately criticized. In 1962, the Chinese population had reached 672.95 million, a net increase of 131.28 million over 1949 when the PRC was founded.[14] Faced with the increasingly serious contradiction between economic and social development and population growth, the Chinese government gradually increased its control efforts. On December 18, 1962, the CPC Central Committee and the State Council issued central authorities' first family planning document – *Instructions on Advocacy of Family Planning*. According to the document, "In cities and densely populated rural areas, we should advocate birth control to properly control the natural growth rate of population and gradually make childbearing a planned practice. This is an established policy in the country's endeavour to develop socialism."[15] Zhou Enlai talked directly about the need to practice family planning in Beijing at the 101st Session of the Standing Committee of the Second National People's Congress in July 1963. He said, "Cities should lead the effort. In the case of Beijing, its population growth rate last year was 3.5 per cent (excluding the outer suburbs). The country's average population growth rate was 2.5 per cent. At the same time, Beijing's was 3.5 per cent, so the population of this city is growing too fast."[16] In September 1963, the CPC Central Committee held the second national conference on cities, which made specific plans for the family planning campaign in cities. It was made clear that "a family planning campaign involving the general public should be launched nationwide. All

---

13 China's population growth stagnated for a short time in the period from 1960 to 1961 when the country suffered economic hardship but rebounded in 1962 due to the remedial childbearing policy.

14 Tian Xueyuan. 2009. *60 Years of China's Population Policy*. Beijing: Social Sciences Academic Press. 103.

15 Party Literature Research Office of the CPC Central Committee, ed. 1997. *Selected Important Documents Since the Founding of the People's Republic of China* (*Volume 15*). Beijing: Central Party Literature Publishing House. 763.

16 Editorial Office of *Family Planning in China*, ed. 1997. *Party and State Leaders' Views on Population and Family Planning: 1950s-70s*. Beijing: China Population Publishing House. 14.

sectors should be involved in the educational and organisational efforts to make the great significance of family planning known to all so that people take the initiative to act."[17] In response to the call of the CPC Central Committee and in light of the city's specific population issues, the Beijing Municipal Government launched a multi-pronged public campaign for family planning.

2.1 *Setting Up Family Planning Organizations at Different Levels*

In January 1963, the CPC Beijing Municipal Committee established the leading group for family planning following the guidelines of the *Instructions on Advocacy of Family Planning* issued by the CPC Central Committee and the State Council. However, "on the whole, family planning was not taken seriously enough, there was a lack of active efforts, and some measures were not implemented".[18] As the city's population kept growing in the first half of 1963, especially after Zhou Enlai's speech in July, the CPC Beijing Municipal Committee decided, in October of the year, to set up a Family Planning Commission led by Wan Li to replace the leading group for family planning. On October 29, 1963, the CPC Beijing Municipal Committee issued an essential directive on family planning, requiring that Party committees at all levels should place family planning as one of the most important items on their agenda to make real progress and all districts and counties should further strengthen their leadership in family planning and establish leading organizations in enterprises, public institutions and government agencies.[19] The directive was then communicated and acted on at the district/country level. Chongwen District set up a family planning committee headed by the district's Party secretary. "The leading groups for family planning of Dongcheng, Xicheng, Xuanwu, Haidian and Shijingshan districts also discussed the municipal Party committee's instructions and proposed establishing a family planning committee. It was suggested that one Party secretary should serve as the director and one deputy district mayor as the deputy director. The number of committee members was also increased to include the heads of various departments of the district Party committee."[20] Enterprises, factories, government agencies and public institutions also improved family planning organizations in a short period. For

17 Peng Peiyun, ed. *Family Planning in China*. Beijing: China Population Publishing House. 6.

18 Leading Group of Beijing Municipality for Family Planning. "Opinions on Advancing Family Planning (Draft)." Beijing Municipal Archives: 002–020-00380.

19 CPC Beijing Municipal Committee. "Opinions of the Leading Group of Beijing Municipality for Family Planning on Advancing Family Planning (October 1963)." Beijing Municipal Archives: 002–020-00380.

20 Office of Beijing Municipal Family Planning Commission. "Family Planning Debriefing (No.1, 1963)." Beijing Municipal Archives: 002–020-00379.

example, Beijing's No.718 Factory established family planning committees or leading groups headed by main leaders at different levels, and their specific responsibilities were clearly defined. "The Party secretary had overall charge of related operations, the administrative department provided support in terms of manpower and time, the trade union was responsible for public education and the sale of contraceptives, the Communist Youth League focused on the education on late marriage, and the health department was responsible for the dissemination of scientific knowledge and technical guidance."[21] In addition, to strengthen leadership, the factory also improved the family planning reporting system and carried out inspections as planned to ensure that all measures were implemented. According to a report published by the Beijing Municipal Family Planning Commission, during this period, "organizations in all districts and counties established leading groups for family planning",[22] which provided an organizational guarantee for advancing related work.

2.2 *Identifying and Training Leading Communication Specialists*

The purpose of the family planning campaign launched by the Beijing Municipal Government was to make family planning known in the city through publicity and education and "significantly increase the number of people supporting the family planning policy on the basis of raising public awareness". Therefore, efforts focused on the training of leading communication specialists.

The Beijing Municipal Family Planning Commission selected people with "a positive mindset, the ability to be close to the general public, and enthusiasm for family planning" as candidates for leading communication specialists.[23] At the local level, however, relevant organizations considered it more important that the candidates "did well in contraception so they could set a good example to others".[24] In addition, leading communication specialists should "have adequate knowledge of family planning, have practised or have the need for contraception, and be trusted by others" because such people would play a role

21 Office of Beijing Municipal Family Planning Commission. "How Beijing 718 Factory Strengthened Leadership to Make Family Planning an Established Practice (March 28, 1964)." Beijing Municipal Archives: 002–020-00391.

22 Office of Beijing Municipal Family Planning Commission. "Report of the Office of Beijing Municipal Family Planning Commission to the Fourth Meeting of the Commission (December 31, 1965)." Beijing Municipal Archives: 002–020-00376.

23 Beijing Municipal Family Planning Commission. "Report on Family Planning (Draft)." Beijing Municipal Archives: 002–020-00391.

24 Office of Beijing Municipal Family Planning Commission. "Some Practices of Jingmian No.2 Factory in Promoting Family Planning (December 21, 1963)." Beijing Municipal Archives: 002–020-00379.

much better than policy communication. In Beijing Jingmian No.2 Factory, for example, "many of the leading communication specialists would talk about their experience in practising contraception ... Thanks to such sharing, more people are now taking the initiative to use birth control".[25]

Then, the selected leading communication specialists were brought together, and training at various levels and of different types was given to them to clarify their thinking and raise their awareness. Special training was organized to address the wrong ideas of some officials that "birth control was not a serious matter", "it was dishonorable", and "even an honor associated with it was not something worth sharing."[26] Firstly, the great significance of family planning was explained in the context of local realities, and it was emphasized that promoting family planning was a worthy cause. "When talking about the benefits of family planning, the focus should be not only on explaining its significance but also on the citation of real examples that people can relate to."[27] Secondly, professionals were invited to explain how fertility works, what contraception is and the use of contraceptives from a medical point of view. Thirdly, when the right ideas and methods were made clear, the leading communication specialists were told what exactly they needed to do and the points for attention.

By December 1965, Beijing had "trained more than a hundred thousand family planning communication specialists".[28] They were quickly involved in the family planning campaign and played a leading role in communicating the policy and setting a good example.

2.3 *Making Meticulous Communication Efforts*

A critical way Beijing organized the family planning campaign was to communicate the right ideas to the general public by holding various meetings first for officials and then for the people. "To make the family planning policy well known to all people", Beijing Jingmian No.2 Factory "first held a general meeting of the management, a general meeting of Party members, a general

---

25 Office of Beijing Municipal Family Planning Commission. "Some Practices of Jingmian No.2 Factory in Promoting Family Planning (December 21, 1963)." Beijing Municipal Archives: 002–020-00379.

26 Beijing Municipal Family Planning Commission. "Some Thoughts on Family Planning." Beijing Municipal Archives: 002–020-00378.

27 Beijing Women's Federation. "How the First Team of Xishan Production Brigade of Sijiqing People's Commune Trained People Active in Promoting Family Planning (June 1963)." Beijing Municipal Archives: 084–002-00295.

28 Office of Beijing Municipal Family Planning Commission. "Report of the Office of Beijing Municipal Family Planning Commission to the Fourth Meeting of the Commission (December 31, 1965)." Beijing Municipal Archives: 002–020-00376.

meeting of Youth League members and a meeting of veteran workers and then employees' meetings workshop by workshop", so that relevant information was communicated to all employees of the factory. Moreover, the factory's leading communication specialists paid visits to employees' homes. They "visited 1,767 households and all of the 148 people who were fertile had heard their report three or four times."[29]

"Comparisons, facts and calculations" and role models were used to inspire the people. The leading communication specialists would compare the past and present pros and cons in communicating the family planning policy. The Lugouqiao People's Commune in Fengtai District, for example, "asked people to talk about the differences between the old society and the new one, the pain of having more children and the benefits of having fewer, their feelings and demands, and the care of the Party for farmers' life ... After three months of communication, more than 2,700 of the 7,900 fertile women in the commune had used intrauterine devices or had other contraceptive operations".[30] At No.1 Branch of Beijing 718 Factory, the leading communication specialists held a meeting with female workers. "Many workers at the meeting talked about how more children would impose a heavy economic burden on the families and consume the energy of their mothers." After comparison, "some concluded that having one child would lead to a reduction in salary by two grades on average and asking a leave in the case of the child getting sick would cause incalculable loss to work and family and that having more children would lead to the lack of drive for doing better at work or pursuing further education."[31] In this way, the significance of birth control was highlighted and communication efforts would be easier to produce results.

The effects of communication were maximised by making models, wall charts and slides, holding exhibitions, screening family planning films, etc. Beijing "printed and distributed more than 600,000 copies of promotional materials and produced several hundred sets of models, wall charts and slides", which stimulated the public's interest and enhanced the effects of communication. For example, members of the Qingyundian Commune "were interested

29 Office of Beijing Municipal Family Planning Commission. "Some Practices of Jingmian No.2 Factory in Promoting Family Planning (December 21, 1963)." Beijing Municipal Archives: 002–020-00379.

30 Office of Beijing Municipal Family Planning Commission. "Report of the Office of Beijing Municipal Family Planning Commission to the Fourth Meeting of the Commission (December 31, 1965)." Beijing Municipal Archives: 002–020-00376.

31 Office of Beijing Municipal Family Planning Commission. "Family Planning Efforts of No.1 Branch of Beijing 718 Factory (December 24, 1963)." Beijing Municipal Archives: 002–020 -00379.

in the knowledge of physical hygiene, and the explanation with pictures and objects was prevalent."[32] The screening of family planning films, as one of the direct approaches adopted by the government, helped to enhance the effectiveness of family planning communication.

Different communication methods were adopted for different groups of people. The Publicity Department of the CPC Beijing Municipal Committee required that "married young and middle-aged people should be encouraged to practice contraception and learn more about family planning; those who had too many children could be given appropriate education about permanent birth control, and unmarried young people should be strongly encouraged to build a career before starting a family".[33] Leading communication specialists well applied the guideline in their day-to-day operations. For example, the leading communication specialists at the Bingmasi Neighborhood Committee of Fengsheng Subdistrict Office in Xicheng District disseminated the knowledge of contraception in a targeted manner. For women in lactation, they emphasized the reason why they could not get pregnant during the lactation period; for those who asked to use a vaginal ring, they explained the effect and benefits of using the device; for those who asked to have a tubal operation, they explained that the procedure would not lead to any sequela. People found this way of communication practical and accessible.[34] All these were verified in the author's visit to Fengsheng Community Neighborhood Committeeof Financial Street Subdistrict Office, Xicheng District.[35] Most people around the community have a strong impression about the family planning campaign of the year. As recalled by the elders, communication efforts were made on a large scale during the campaign and family planning would be a topic at meetings held at their workplaces.[36]

---

32 Office of Beijing Municipal Family Planning Commission. "Family Planning Debriefing (No.11, 1964)." Beijing Municipal Archives: 002–020-00391.

33 Publicity Department of the CPC Beijing Municipal Committee. "Several Problems Needing Attention in the Communication of Family Planning Policy among the Public (December 27, 1963)." Beijing Municipal Archives: 001–012-00575.

34 Office of Beijing Municipal Family Planning Commission. "Some Experience of Bingmasi Neighborhood Committee of Fengsheng Subdistrict Office in Xicheng District in Promoting Family Planning (December 26, 1963)." Beijing Municipal Archives: 002–020-00379.

35 Due to the change of times and the adjustment of zoning, Fengsheng Subdistrict Office has been merged with the Financial Street Subdistrict Office, and the former has been renamed Fengsheng Neighborhood Committee. Then Bingmasi Neighborhood Committee and Fengsheng Neighborhood Committee merged to form a new Fengsheng Community Neighborhood Committee.

36 Based on an interview conducted by the author in Fengsheng Community, Financial Street Subdistrict Office, Xicheng District, Beijing on July 31, 2013, with senior citizens LF (84), CH (70) and ZY (78).

2.4 *Providing Technical Support for Birth Control*

In the second half of 1963, Wan Li, Director of Beijing Municipal Family Planning Commission, said at the meeting of district and county family planning committee directors, "We should still focus on advocating late marriage and contraception."[37] Relevant departments made further requirement that "intensified efforts should be made to encourage contraception", and that "couples with more children should be encouraged to have a tubal operation on a voluntary basis and the quality of the operation should be ensured".[38] In fact, at that time, the supply of contraceptives and related medical facilities in Beijing was far from enough to meet the needs of the family planning campaign, and even some medical professionals lacked knowledge about family planning. "It was widely reported that many medical workers did not have enough knowledge of contraception, especially those who had just graduated from universities. They had learned little in school and knew only a few simple methods. Veteran ones had no experience in this regard, so they did not know much about it either."[39] In response to these problems, Beijing accelerated the development of an online platform for family planning, which provided technical support for related efforts.

A sales network for contraceptives was formed. Firstly, in February 1963, the Beijing Municipal Public Health Bureau and other authorities issued the Joint Circular on Strengthening Contraceptive Supply and the Circular on Agency Sale of Contraceptives by Medical Institutions.[40] As required by the circular, relevant organizations made efforts to produce birth control drugs and instruments of "good quality, wide variety, complete specifications and sufficient quantity" to meet the market supply. "Medical and commercial departments, rural supply and marketing cooperatives, shops and medical institutions at all levels in Beijing set up outlets to sell products and offer instructions to people on how to use them. At the end of 1963, a contraceptives sales network covering urban and rural areas took shape in Beijing."[41] "In 1964, more than

37 "Minutes of Meeting of District and County Family Planning Committee Directors Held by Beijing Municipal Family Planning Commission (December 13, 1963)." Beijing Municipal Archives: 002–020-00378.

38 Editorial Committee of *Beijing Gazetteer*, ed. 2004. *Annals of Beijing: Population*. Beijing: Beijing Publishing House. 261.

39 Office of Beijing Municipal Family Planning Commission. "Family Planning Debriefing (No.3, 1963)." Beijing Municipal Archives: 002–020-00379.

40 Editorial Committee of *Beijing Gazetteer*, ed. 2004. *Annals of Beijing: Population*. Beijing: Beijing Publishing House. 268.

41 Editorial Committee of *Beijing Gazetteer*, ed. 2004. *Annals of Beijing: Population*. Beijing: Beijing Publishing House. 268.

7.7 million condoms were sold in the city, an increase of seventy-one per cent over 1962 when family planning was not widely carried out, and an increase of ten per cent over 1963."[42] The sales outlets were said to be very popular the general public. For example, the clinic of Beijing Low Voltage Electrical Appliances Factory began selling contraceptives on November 21, 1963. They even introduced a door-to-door delivery service, which was applauded by local residents. "They said that it was more convenient than going to the store, and in the three days from November 21 to 23" contraceptives were even out of stock.[43] Secondly, contraceptive drugs and related medical expenses were included in the employment security system, and the expenses arising from family planning would be reduced or fully covered by the government. According to relevant regulations, for example, "employees and the family members enjoying employment security would be exempted from paying for contraception clinic service, use of diaphragm, and tubal operation. Urban residents and rural commune members might be exempt according to the specific circumstances. Those working for the government would be paid as usual and still qualified for performance-based awards despite a leave for contraception-related matters."[44]

A medical technology network was established. Firstly, the medical sector worked hard to improve medical services for family planning. In response to the shortage of beds for tubal operations, Beijing made a plan to "set up outpatient clinics for offering family planning guidance in urban medical institutions, increasing outpatient service time and the number of beds for tubal operations, and simplifying procedures".[45] Facing the problems of medical professionals' "impatience", insufficient knowledge of contraception and "incomplete mastery of technology,"[46] medical sector strengthened education and training for doctors, increased oversight over service providers, and encouraged them to learn from international practices, to reduce the incidence of errors

42 Beijing Municipal Archives and Party History Research Office of the CPC Beijing Municipal Committee, ed. 2007. *Selected Important Documents of Beijing (1965)*. Beijing: China Archives Publishing House. 315.

43 Office of Beijing Municipal Family Planning Commission. "Family Planning Debriefing (No.7, 1963)." Beijing Municipal Archives: 002–020-00379.

44 Office of Beijing Municipal Family Planning Commission. "Report of the Office of Beijing Municipal Family Planning Commission to the Fourth Meeting of the Commission (December 31, 1965)." Beijing Municipal Archives: 002–020-00376.

45 Li Xugang. "A Report on Family Planning to the CPC Beijing Municipal Committee." Beijing Municipal Archives: 002–020-00391.

46 Office of Beijing Municipal Family Planning Commission. "Family Planning Debriefing (No.3, 1963)." Beijing Municipal Archives: 002–020-00379.

and accidents. Community-level health centers and clinics also followed the example of municipal and district medical institutions to improve family planning services. For instance, under the guidance of the health station, the clinic of Beijing 718 Factory organized lectures on family planning to educate workers on birth control methods.[47] Through study sessions, Qingyundian Commune Health Center learned how to operate intrauterine contraceptive device placement. Before the family planning campaign, commune members would often visit large hospitals for contraception, which was a waste of manpower and financial resources. After the commune health center had obtained relevant equipment, people said that "it would be much better if the service were available earlier."[48] Secondly, medical teams were sent to rural areas to provide birth control-related drugs and services for local residents. They disseminated scientific knowledge and methods of contraception, performed intrauterine contraceptive device placement, induced abortion and vasectomy operations, and trained local medical personnel, which eliminated blind spots in the family planning medical network and delivered convenience to rural residents. The medical teams even changed their service routine to meet the contraception needs of women in remote areas. "They worked around the clock. People did not need to make any appointments or registrations and would have an operation immediately after an examination by a medical team member."[49] It was very popular among local people. For example, "nine women had operations for intrauterine contraceptive device placement in Qingyangtun Production Brigade of Menlou Village Commune during the period when the medical team was stationed in Menlou Village, and after the medical team moved to Mafang Commune, another twenty-one women asked to have the same operation."[50] The provision of related services and the supply of contraceptive drugs and tools kept up with needs. "Local people had access to convenient services, and medical personnel's serving rural residents helped to extend the positive influence of the health workforce." As the CPC Beijing Municipal Committee

47 Office of Beijing Municipal Family Planning Commission. "How Beijing 718 Factory Strengthened Leadership to Make Family Planning an Established Practice (March 28, 1964)." Beijing Municipal Archives: 002–020-00391.

48 Office of Beijing Municipal Family Planning Commission. "Family Planning Debriefing (No.6, 1963)." Beijing Municipal Archives: 002–020-00379.

49 Office of Beijing Municipal Family Planning Commission. "Trial Operation of Medical Teams in Sanluju Production Brigade of Lugouqiao Commune (March 31, 1964)." Beijing Municipal Archives: 002–020-00391.

50 Office of Beijing Municipal Family Planning Commission. "Family Planning Debriefing (No.7, 1964)." Beijing Municipal Archives: 002–020-00391.

said in a document submitted to the CPC Central Committee, "This ensured smooth progress in carrying out related work."[51]

3 The Effects of Family Planning Campaign in Beijing

After more than two years of efforts, the Beijing Municipal Family Planning Commission concluded that the city's family planning campaign "achieved great progress and remarkable results", thanks to strong leadership, training of leading players, large-scale communication and the application of medical technology. Firstly, the birth rate was reduced. "In 1964, more than 229,000 people were born in the city, a decrease of 89,000 over 1963, and the birth rate dropped from 43.4 births per thousand people to 30.4 births per thousand people. From January to September 1965, more than 132,000 people were born in the city, some 41,000 fewer than that in the same period of 1964. For the whole year, there would be probably more than 180,000 newborns, and the birth rate would drop to around twenty-three births per thousand people."[52] Secondly, "the family planning policy basically became well-known and it was well accepted by many people", starting to exert profound influence.[53] However, in the early days of the campaign, there were some improper practices. For example, in November 1963, the first month when the city began to launch the large-scale family planning campaign, the number of couples married at a registry in Beijing hit a record high. "A total of ninety-six couples registered for marriage from November 1 to 21, an increase of forty pairs or 71.4 per cent over the same period of October, according to Qianmen, Donghua, Tiyuguanlu and Chongwai offices."[54] According to the analysis of the Beijing Municipal People's Committee, this was because people were concerned about restrictions on late marriage and childbearing following the implementation of family planning policy. According to the investigation of People's Committee members in 1964,

51 Beijing Municipal Archives and Party History Research Office of the CPC Beijing Municipal Committee, ed. 2007. *Selected Important Documents of Beijing (1965)*. Beijing: China Archives Publishing House. 315.

52 Office of Beijing Municipal Family Planning Commission. "Report of the Office of Beijing Municipal Family Planning Commission to the Fourth Meeting of the Commission (December 31, 1965)." Beijing Municipal Archives: 002–020-00376.

53 Beijing Municipal Archives and Party History Research Office of the CPC Beijing Municipal Committee, ed. 2007. *Selected Important Documents of Beijing (1965)*. Beijing: China Archives Publishing House. 312.

54 General Office of the People's Committee of Beijing Municipality. "Debriefing (November 29, 1963)." Beijing Municipal Archives: 002–020-00377.

some married people still "valued sons over daughters" and the unmarried ones were still "afraid that the *Marriage Law* would be amended and thus anxious to register for getting married."[55] In such a context, some organizations made hard and fast rules that must be enforced. In May 1964, a young man in Fengtai District "reported that some practices in promoting birth control were not appropriate" in an anonymous letter, which disclosed that his employer required that "employees who did not get married as required would be punished with dismissal or public criticism".[56] In this regard, the Beijing Municipal Family Planning Commission stressed that "people should be encouraged to pursue the policy on a voluntary basis but not forced to do so, saying "we have made it clear from the very beginning that we should not ask people to make plans and promise anything, set specific targets for them to reach, or try to promote family planning through competition".[57] This requirement reversed the mandatory practices of some organizations in the early days of the campaign. Materials available show that from the policy guidelines to the grassroots practice, this family planning campaign was mainly advanced through communication and education, and there are very few mandatory practices.

The family planning campaign led to a rapid decrease in the natural growth rate of Beijing's population. There are mainly three main factors that contributed to the decline. The first one is the communication and education efforts during this period. The communication efforts made the family planning policy a government initiative. The education efforts made people realize for the first time that family planning could be connected with national interest and personal life, giving this new policy ethical justification and initially winning popular support for the campaign. The second one is the large-scale supply of birth control products is more critical. In this campaign, the Beijing Municipal Government put into market a large number of birth control devices to ease the shortage of such products and thus meet people's needs in this regard, which slowed down population growth in the short term. The third one is the support of policies related to the family planning campaign and the training of medical professionals. After the family planning campaign began, Party and government departments at all levels in Beijing strengthened their leadership over efforts to promote birth control. In addition, a series of regulations were

55 Office of Beijing Municipal Family Planning Commission. "Family Planning Debriefing (No.5, 1964)." Beijing Municipal Archives: 002–020-00391.

56 General Office of the People's Committee of Beijing Municipality. "Debriefing (May 25, 1964)." Beijing Municipal Archives: 002–020-00377.

57 Li Xugang. "A Report on Family Planning to the CPC Beijing Municipal Committee." Beijing Municipal Archives: 002–020-00391.

issued concerning visit to a birth control clinic, leave for induced abortion, salary matters and the extent of expense reduction and reimbursement for tubal operation. Medical professionals went to rural areas to "disseminate knowledge of birth control, perform tubal operations, and helped to train the technical backbone of family planning in communes and production brigades, leading to a sharp decline in the number of newborns in Beijing for several consecutive years".[58] The CPC Beijing Municipal Committee attributed the success of efforts in this phase firstly to "the instructions of the CPC Central Committee and the State Council on advocating family planning which were in the immediate interests and requirements of the general public".[59] This is indeed a real reason that fits the situation at the time. It should be noted, however, that the main beneficiaries of these technologies were those who had already given birth to a second or third child or who did not want to have more children because of financial burden, as well as young people who had decided to delay pregnancy as a result of education activities. They became the main contributors to the slowdown in population growth during this period. However, the contribution of these people is limited after all. At the end of 1965, as the family planning campaign continued, "more people were married in the year compared with 1964, the average age became a little younger, and the proportion of first and second births increased."[60] The Beijing Municipal Government held that to curb the rapid population growth was a "great challenge that needed to be addressed in the long term",[29](p. 317) and more people should be encouraged to support family planning voluntarily. Beijing's family planning campaign was interrupted when the Cultural Revolution started, but the people, especially urban residents, had developed a preliminary understanding of the family planning policy.

---

58 Editorial Committee of *Beijing Gazetteer*, ed. 2004. *Annals of Beijing: Population*. Beijing: Beijing Publishing House. 247.

59 Beijing Municipal Archives and Party History Research Office of the CPC Beijing Municipal Committee, ed. 2007. *Selected Important Documents of Beijing (1965)*. Beijing: China Archives Publishing House. 313.

60 Office of Beijing Municipal Family Planning Commission. "Report of the Office of Beijing Municipal Family Planning Commission to the Fourth Meeting of the Commission (December 31, 1965)." Beijing Municipal Archives: 002–020-00376.

CHAPTER 13

A Study on the Rural Medical Practitioner Training Model in the First 30 Years of the People's Republic of China

*Li Decheng**

Abstract

When the People's Republic of China was founded, there was a serious shortage of medical services and medicines in rural areas. The Communist Party of China and the Chinese government kept introducing institutional innovation and offered training to millions of rural medical practitioners in a short period of time, who provided basic medical services for rural residents. The establishment of such a training model with Chinese characteristics made the country well-adapted to the development of rural medical care, setting an example for other developing countries to address their medical care problems.

Keywords

People's Republic of China – rural areas – medical practitioners – primary level – cooperative medical care

After[1] the founding of the People's Republic of China (PRC), the Communist Party of China (CPC) and the Chinese government strived to build a medical care system with Chinese characteristics in rural areas to solve the severe shortage of medical services and medicines there. In the 1950s, they began to use the rich human resources in rural areas to train medical practitioners in

* Li Decheng, Ph.D. in history, is an associate professor at the School of History, Culture and Tourism, Jiangxi Normal University.

1 This paper is an outcome of the key research project "A Study on Traditional Cooperative Medical Care and Barefoot Doctors in Rural China" (07ZD010) included in Jiangxi Province's Education and Science Plan, which is also a project of provincial key research base of Humanities and Social Sciences carried out through open tender.

 | DOI:10.1163/9789004737990_014

a well-planned way. In the early 1980s, a brand-new medical care system was established in rural China.

1 Establishment of Medical Care System in the Early Years of the People's Republic of China

Earth-shaking changes have occurred in Chinese society over the past 60 years since the founding of the PRC. The CPC has led the Chinese people on the path of building and developing socialism with Chinese characteristics, creating one great miracle after another. In particular, the introduction of cooperative medical care and the training of rural medical practitioners on a large scale have been recognized by some foreign experts as the "China model" for solving rural medical care problems in developing countries. This model played a significant role in alleviating the severe shortage of medical services and medicines in rural areas, increasing the accessibility of primary healthcare services to rural residents, and improving the health of the rural population, for which it was widely acclaimed. This "China model" was created in a country with a weak economy. Millions of rural medical practitioners were trained in a short period, on a large scale, at a low cost and with high efficiency to solve the problem of meeting the basic healthcare needs of a massive population in vast rural areas. It was a unique achievement in world history, for which the WHO considers it "the only good example of health financing in developing countries".[2] It has also been hailed as a successful "health revolution".[3] This model was created under the leadership of the CPC when the country acquired extraordinary resilience thanks to the continued promotion of institutional and policy innovation and the creation of an enabling institutional framework for social development and national rejuvenation.

In 1949, China faced economic depression, heavy social crises, underdevelopment of science, culture and healthcare, and low living standards. Infectious, parasitic and endemic diseases were prevalent, but healthcare resources were very scarce. At the time, there were only 505,040 practitioners of traditional Chinese medicine (TCM) and Western medicine in China, accounting for only 0.92 permille of the country's total population. There were only 2,600 hospitals with eighty thousand beds (0.15 beds per thousand people on average) in the

2 Chen Jiagui. 2001. *Report on the Development of Social Security in China*. Beijing: Social Sciences Academic Press. 280.

3 World Bank. 1994. *China: Long-term Problems in the Transformation of Healthcare Model and Countermeasures*. Beijing: China Financial and Economic Publishing House. 17.

country, and only 20,133 beds were in rural areas, whose residents accounted for more than eighty-five per cent of the national populations. According to the statistics for 1947, there were only 1,437 county hospitals in China, all of which were ill-equipped. Each hospital had an average of more than ten beds and very few medical facilities. There were even fewer medical institutions in villages and towns. Moreover, there was a severe shortage of medicines, most of which could not be produced domestically. Even the most straightforward medical instruments had to be imported.[4] The limited healthcare resources were far from meeting people's needs for disease prevention and treatment. In the vast rural areas, there were few medical practitioners except for a small number of TCM doctors who were mainly concentrated in market towns or places where transportation was relatively developed. In the rural areas with inconvenient transportation and scattered residences, the lack of medical services and medicine was even more severe, so it was urgent to establish primary-level medical institutions.

In the face of this situation, China must develop a nationwide medical care system to address the urgent shortage of medical services and medicines for the people effectively. But what kind of system should be designed to effectively solve the healthcare problem of a country which had a large population and a weak economy at the time? China chose a medical care model different from that of Western countries and developed an innovative public health system with Chinese characteristics. The system was characterized by the reliance on low-skilled medical workers trained in a short period of time, the development of labor-intensive rather than capital-intensive medical techniques, the emphasis on prevention and primary healthcare, and the focus on public health programs rather than solely on the health of individuals. In the 1950s, China started the endeavor to train rural medical practitioners using the rich human resources in the countryside and established a brand-new medical care system that connected rural medical workers with their counterparts on a higher level and those in the cities, leading to the continued improvement of their medical techniques.

2 Training Model of Rural Medical Practitioners before the Wide Application of Cooperative Medical Care

To address the lack of medical services and medicines in rural areas, the CPC and the Chinese government introduced the health policy of "serving the vast

4 Beijing University of Chinese Medicine, ed. 1978. *A History of Chinese Medicine.* Shanghai: Shanghai Scientific and Technical Publishers. 62.

majority of the people, focusing more on preventive measures, utilizing both Western medicine and TCM, and incorporating health promotion and people's involvement". Under this guidance of this policy, the government launched a nationwide Patriotic Hygiene campaign, in conjunction with the efforts to promote disease prevention, and sent health workers to investigate local realities about infectious diseases and formulate disease prevention plans. Before disease prevention plans were implemented, a rural medical care system had to be established which would require the training of medical practitioners to expand the staffing of primary-level medical institutions. In the early 1950s, the central government planned for the training of rural medical workers to alleviate the shortage of healthcare resources. In 1951, the Ministry of Health issued the *Specific Measures for Developing Primary-level Medical Institutions in Rural Areas* (*Draft*). According to the document, the plan for 1951 was to train many medical workers to develop primary-level medical institutions gradually. Primary-level medical workers were divided into health workers, maternal and child healthcare workers (midwives), and nurse assistants. It is suggested that "health workers should be selected from workers, farmers and primary school teachers (including rural primary school teachers and students in private schools)" while "maternal and child healthcare workers and nurse assistants should be selected from rural traditional midwives, factory girls, rural women and primary school teachers". The selected candidates should be "given on-the-job training for a short period of time". Specifically, "health workers should be trained by district-level health clinics (or county health centers) while maternal and child healthcare workers and nurse assistants should be trained by county health centers."[5] Moreover, the timetable for training was devised; nurse assistants and maternal and child healthcare workers would receive training for half a year while health workers for eight weeks.

In the early 1950s, as required by the central government, the first primary-level medical workers in rural areas were trained in a short period of time. Local health institutions selected rural youths for on-site training. Take Shengxian County of Zhejiang Province as an example. From November 29, 1954, to January 16, 1955, a training session for rural health workers was held on a trial basis in Guandi Village, Xibei Township. A total of 26 persons were given training on epidemic prevention, first aid and maternal and child healthcare. In early February 1955, a five-day training program was conducted in Chengguan and Chongren, with a total of 1,100 rural health workers trained. Training courses included schistosomiasis, trauma first aid, epidemic prevention knowledge, and maternal and child healthcare. In November of the same year, 203 health

5 Department of Community-level Healthcare and MCH, Ministry of Health, ed. *Collection of Documents on Rural Healthcare* (*1951–2000*). 247–248.

workers were trained in two separate sessions.[6] With the advancement of rural health promotion efforts, the government set up primary-level medical institutions in rural areas one after another. By 1958, county hospitals had been set up in almost all counties; after 1958, commune clinics began to be established and the shortage of rural healthcare resources was eased. On April 15, 1959, the Ministry of Health issued *Several Opinions on Strengthening the Healthcare Services of People's Communes*, proposing the training of health workers, child-care workers, cooks and birth attendants in rural areas. It was pointed out that "the selected candidates for health workers, child-care workers and birth attendants should cover a wide range of ages".[7] To strengthen the management of rural medical institutions and the training of rural medical workers in the context of the gradual establishment of a preventive care system in rural areas, in 1962, the Ministry of Health issued the *Opinions on Several Issues Concerning Improving Hospital Operations* (*Draft*), which required that "county hospitals should provide technical guidance to rural medical institutions in a planned and focused way".[8] In 1965, the Department of Medical Education of the Ministry of Health issued to health departments and bureaus of provinces, municipalities and autonomous regions and forty-one medical colleges and universities the *Opinions on Further Strengthening the On-the-job Training of Rural Health Workers and Birth Attendants*. It is proposed that "within three to five years from 1965 efforts should be made to ensure that every production brigade had birth attendants and every production team had health workers". After training, the health workers should have abilities in three aspects: first, the ability to identify twenty to thirty local common diseases, deal with minor injuries and diseases common in rural production and life, provide simple first-aid support, and use common drugs and simple acupuncture treatment methods; second, the ability to employ the methods of eliminating the "four pests", manage water and excrement sanitation, and apply the knowledge of organizing patriotic sanitation campaigns and public health education activities; third, the ability to report epidemic outbreaks and take simple measures to prevent infectious diseases (such as prophylactic injection). Birth attendants should be trained to be able to employ new delivery methods, conduct antenatal examinations, provide simple care for mothers and newborns, promote education on family planning, place pessaries and guide the placement

6 *Health Annals of Shengxian County* (internal issue), February 1987.179.

7 Department of Community-level Healthcare and MCH, Ministry of Health, ed. *Collection of Documents on Rural Healthcare* (*1951–2000*). 9–10.

8 Department of Community-level Healthcare and MCH, Ministry of Health, ed. *Collection of Documents on Rural Healthcare* (*1951–2000*). 265.

of vaginal septa.[9] This detailed document provided effective guidance for the training of rural medical workers.

On June 26, 1965, Mao Zedong issued a directive about "putting the focus of healthcare promotion on rural areas". After that, intensified efforts were made for the training of medical workers in rural areas. For example, by 1966, 1,331 health workers had been trained in the four counties of Zhoushan, Zhejiang, by combining centralized training with the guidance of production teams. After that, further training was provided in the principle of offering what was needed.[10] In September, the central government approved the report of the Party Committee of the Ministry of Health on putting the focus of healthcare promotion on rural areas. It was stressed again that "great efforts should be made to train medical workers for rural areas and offer on-the-job training for medical workers in production teams and production brigades to equip communes' health institutions with four to five doctors of better quality". The nature, tasks and training methods of rural medical workers were also specified. "Part-time medical practitioners should be health workers in production teams and farmer-doctors in production brigades. Health workers should be able to practice acupuncture, treat common minor injuries and diseases, and offer preventive care and first-aid support." "Training could be provided by rural medical teams and local health institutions, or by offering healthcare classes in agricultural secondary schools. Farmer-doctors in production brigades could be trained in slack seasons for two or three consecutive years." "Political thinking should be valued in the selection and training of all medical workers."[11] In line with the guiding principle of this report, the large-scale training of rural health workers began nationwide in 1966.

In the mid-1960s, the training of rural health workers began to be organized on different levels with the development of rural cooperative medical care and the establishment of a three-tiered preventive care network. One was the training of health workers in production teams, and the other was the training of health workers in production brigades. Health workers were selected from medical workers who had done a good job in offering healthcare and then trained to acquire knowledge of several or more than a dozen common diseases in rural areas and the skills for giving first-aid treatment before taking

9 Zhang, Kaining, ed. 2002. *From Barefoot Doctors to Village Doctors*. Kunming: Yunnan People's Publishing House. 17.

10 "Report of the Health Bureau of Zhoushan Commissioner's Office in Zhejiang Province on Health Workers' Activities (May 30, 1966)." Zhejiang Archives: J165-16-81.

11 Department of Community-level Healthcare and MCH, Ministry of Health, ed. *Collection of Documents on Rural Healthcare (1951–2000)*. 29–30.

on healthcare tasks of production brigades. They were mainly responsible for treating major common diseases and infectious diseases, offering first aid and arranging for transfer to hospitals, regularly reporting the healthcare efforts of production brigades to commune health centers or county hospitals and receiving their guidance and training.

In 1960, the health authorities in rural areas began to organize medical workers to carry out large-scale vaccination for rural residents, which significantly reduced the incidence of infectious diseases.[12] To consolidate the result, in January 1965, the Ministry of Health issued a circular on issues concerning the organization of mobile medical teams in rural areas. According to the circular, one task of mobile medical teams was to provide medical services in coordination with the socialist education campaign, treating diseases for farmers, especially the poor and lower-middle ones; the other was to offer on-the-job training to health workers and birth attendants of production teams and enhance technical guidance and training for primary-level medical institutions.[13] In February, the Ministry of Health issued the *Circular on Organizing Mobile Medical Teams of Cities for Going to Rural Areas*, stressing again that "a central task of mobile medical teams was to train health workers in rural areas". The Ministry of Health required the mobile medical teams to strengthen the selection and training of rural medical workers leveraging their technical advantages. Therefore, when the medical teams were providing medical services for farmers, they also selected some young farmers for short-term training.[14] Take the training efforts of the No.2 Branch of the Second Medical Team of Hangzhou as an example. With the assistance of local communes and production brigades, the team selected a group of 18-year-old children from poor and lower-middle farmers for short-term training. The training covered physiological anatomy, pathological knowledge, common diseases and drugs, epidemic prevention and hygiene, trauma treatment, first aid in the field, acupuncture and moxibustion, simple care operation, family planning, etc. Each training session would last two months in total, including twenty days of classes followed by practice. During their five-month service in the countryside, 165 health workers were trained for four communes and one

12 C. C. Chen. 1998. *Medicine in Rural China: A Personal Account.* Chengdu: Sichuan People's Publishing House. 142.

13 Department of Community-level Healthcare and MCH, Ministry of Health, ed. *Collection of Documents on Rural Healthcare (1951–2000)*. 620.

14 Department of Community-level Healthcare and MCH, Ministry of Health, ed. *Collection of Documents on Rural Healthcare (1951–2000)*. 627.

town.[15] Another medical team, the Zhejiang Rural Healthcare Promotion Pilot Task Force, provided training for farmer-doctors on a total of eleven subjects including human body structure and physiology, microorganisms, commonly used drugs, medical technology, rural healthcare (including management of parasitic diseases and infectious diseases), surgery, acupuncture, skin diseases, maternal and child healthcare, family planning, trauma, and first aid. The trainees also learned methods of preventing and treating sixty-eight common diseases and fifteen diagnosis and treatment techniques, mastered the application of more than sixty acupuncture points, more than seventy Western medicines and fifty-seven Chinese herbal medicines, and engaged in practical disease prevention and control work.[16] The selection of rural health workers at this stage focused not only on social class of candidates but also on their basic education, and training covered a wide range of subjects. This "general practitioner" training model was beneficial to the growth of health workers, many of whom became barefoot doctors during the cooperative medical care period.

3 Training Model of Rural Barefoot Doctors Following the Wide Application of Cooperative Medical Care

The Ministry of Health originally aimed to reach a certain scale of rural medical workers through five to ten years of training, which means it would take a long time for them to acquire more medical knowledge so that they could better serve the farmers. However, in view of the suffering of farmers and the limited health resources of the country, Mao Zedong decided to intensify the training efforts. The purpose was that they could treat some minor injuries and diseases and relieve the shortage of medical services in rural areas. In addition, remedial measures could be taken and local training could be provided to help them improve in practice. He said, "Medical education should be reformed. The candidates are not necessarily well-educated ... They do not have to be graduates of senior or junior middle schools. Primary school education is enough. They can improve skills in practice. Such doctors may not be able to do something big in rural areas but are better than cheating or witch doctors. It is also economically feasible in the countryside ... The focus of healthcare

15 No.2 Branch of the Second Medical Team in Hangzhou. "Summary Report on the Training On-the-job Health Workers (October 19, 1965)." Zhejiang Archives: J165-15-78.

16 Pilot Team for Rural Healthcare Development in Zhejiang Province. "Preliminary Experience Gained in the First Stage of Farmer-doctor Training (May 21, 1966)." Zhejiang Archives: J165-16-47.

promotion should be put on the rural areas."[17] On the one hand, this view pointed out that medical education at the time did not fit the development of rural medical care, and had an important impact on the medical care efforts in the later stage. It was a turning point in the reform of the country's rural medical care system. On the other hand, it had a great impact on officials and medical workers in the health system at the time. Later on, many urban medical workers were sent to the countryside to receive "re-education" from the poor and lower-middle farmers, producing negative influence on healthcare promotion efforts as a whole.

The approach to the training of rural medical workers changed significantly, with the issuance of Mao Zedong's June 26 directive, especially after the publication of an investigation report on barefoot doctors of Jiangzhen Commune in the suburbs of Shanghai on the *Hongqi* magazine in 1968. According to the report, medical education must be reformed and the Western model should not be adopted anymore; medical colleges and universities should recruit students from barefoot doctors and rural health workers and the training efforts should address the demand for rural health services in one to three years; the quality of services should be improved on the basis of increasing the availability of medical services so that everyone had access to medical care, not just urban residents. A more flexible approach should be adopted for the training of barefoot doctors.[18] After that, the training of rural medical workers was organized on a larger scale and at a higher speed. Rural medical workers became known as "barefoot doctors".

On December 5, 1968, *The People's Daily* reported the practice of the poor and lower-middle farmers' introducing cooperative medical care in Leyuan Commune of Tujia Autonomous County in Changyang, Hubei Province. After that, cooperative medical care began to be promoted nationwide. Most production brigades in the country established cooperative medical care stations, and a nationwide rural medical care system was basically established. Barefoot doctors were primary-level medical workers; their selection, management and training were all included in the cooperative medical care system.

Amid the rise of cooperative medical care, the scale and speed of barefoot doctors' training were increased to solve the problem of insufficient medical workers in rural areas. Take Jiangxi Province as an example. To response to the central government's call, the Revolutionary Committee of Jiangxi Province

---

17 Zhang Kaining, ed. 2002. *From Barefoot Doctors to Village Doctors*. Kunming: Yunnan People's Publishing House. 18.

18 Author unknown. 1968. "The Direction of Medical Education Revolution Seen from the Growth of Barefoot Doctors: An Investigation Report of Shanghai." *Hongqi* 3.

issued the *Decision on Vigorously Training Barefoot Doctors* in early 1969, requiring that "150,000 barefoot doctors should be trained within two years and a rural health service network should be created to completely change healthcare in the province's rural areas". A training plan was also drawn up. "In 1969, sixty thousand to eighty thousand people would be trained, six to seven barefoot doctors in each production brigade, medical service groups would be formed, rural health service network would be established, and cooperative medical care was fully practiced." Although the focus of training was still on the prevention and treatment of common, frequently occurring, infectious and endemic diseases in rural areas, ideological and political education was placed in an important position. It was also required that "the content of training should be adapted to local conditions and cover both TCM and Western medicine, and medical care, preventive care and medicine production should be integrated." Moreover, "barefoot doctors should acquire the hygiene knowledge for building sanitary villages, the knowledge of managing water, excrement and canteens and killing mosquitoes, flies, rats and snails, general birth control techniques, and delivery techniques, master the techniques of preventing and treating local common diseases, frequently-occurring diseases and schistosomiasis, and employ acupuncture, herbal medicines, and folk remedies. They should draw upon and carry forward the medical heritage of the Chinese nation and play a key part in developing new medicine in China." On-site training was combined with farming activities, and training time was greatly shortened. "Barefoot doctors were trained mainly at the primary level. Training classes might be offered in communes or production brigades, or they might be instructed individually. Concentrated training sessions would be held for about three months, mostly in the slack season."[19] Under the guidance of the decision, Jiangxi Province carried out large-scale training of barefoot doctors. By the end of 1975, there were 67,679 health workers and 28,842 birth attendants in production teams across the province.[20] Party organizations and health authorities at all levels attached great importance to the training and education of barefoot doctors and had them well-managed on both political thinking and service fronts. They would be organized to study the theory of the dictatorship of the proletariat as well as the CPC's basic line and encouraged to be Party and Youth League members. In addition, colleges or medical schools

19 Revolutionary Committee of Jiangxi Province. "Decision on Intensifying Efforts to Train Barefoot Doctors." Jiangxi Archives: X032-2-059.

20 "Progress on the Promotion of Cooperative Medical Care and Training of Barefoot Doctors in Jiangxi Province in 1975," in Health Bureau of Jiangxi Province, ed. *Debriefing* 2. Jiangxi Archives: X111-1976Y-005.

and short-term training sessions would be introduced for barefoot doctors, who would have shifts like medical professionals, and medical teams would help improve their skills.[21]

The criteria for the selection of barefoot doctors were basically the same in all parts of the country at the time. They should have a good family background, a passion for the countryside and a willingness to serve the poor and lower-middle farmers. Training was provided locally most of the time, which means concentrated training for a period of time followed repeated training sessions in phases.

Along with the development of cooperative medical care, local teams gathered rich training experience and began to look for new training approaches. Some introduced college classes for barefoot doctors while others started to offer correspondence classes. For example, "in cooperation with suburban county and related hospitals, Beijing No. 2 Hospital launched four college classes for barefoot doctors in rural areas. A total of 205 barefoot doctors with more than three to five years of experience in medical practice were enrolled in the four classes. Faculty members were teachers and clinicians from No.2 Hospital, Friendship Hospital, Workers, Farmers and Soldiers Hospital, Xuanwu Hospital and Chaoyang Hospital."[22] After graduation, all the students returned to their production brigades as barefoot doctors. "In 1973, the University of Barefoot Doctors was established in Yichun, Jiangxi Province with 150 students enrolled. In 1974, the Jiangxi College of Traditional Chinese Medicine resumed correspondence courses on TCM. In the first program, more than four thousand barefoot doctors were enrolled, and in the second one, more than six thousand were enrolled."[23] The training of barefoot doctors continued until the early 1980s. In March 1980, the Ministry of Health issued the *Opinions on Doing Well in the Reform and Development of Healthcare System in One-third of Counties*, requiring that cooperative medical care stations of production brigades should have systematic training so that their barefoot doctors would reach the proficiency of technical secondary school graduates and the team should remain relatively stable". "Existing medical institutions should serve as practice bases, barefoot doctors should be systematically trained and

21 "Development of Barefoot Doctors and Cooperative Medical Care Amid Challenges," in Health Bureau of Jiangxi Province, ed. *Debriefing* (June 14, 1976). Jiangxi Archives: X111-1976Y-005.

22 "Local Health Revolution Practices Introduced in the Health Revolution Debriefing of the Ministry of Health," in Health Bureau of Jiangxi Province, ed. *Debriefing* 4 (March 25, 1976). Jiangxi Archives: X111-1976Y-005.

23 "Introduction to the Utilization of Herbal Medicine in the Development of Cooperative Medical Care in Jiangxi Province (1976)." Jiangxi Archives: X111-1976Y-008.

on-the-job training courses for primary and middle-level medical practitioners should be offered in accordance with the teaching syllabus." The purpose was to ensure that "barefoot doctors could use both TCM and Western medicine to prevent and treat common diseases, do debridement and suturing for wounds, offer first-aid treatment, and provide basic technical guidance on family planning, maternal and child healthcare, etc. and that women doctors could employ new delivery methods."[24] Through extensive and continuous training, a contingent of one million barefoot doctors was developed in a short period. When cooperative medical care was in its prime, there were more than five million rural medical workers in China, including 1.8 million barefoot doctors, 3.5 million health workers and more than 700,000 birth attendants. The size of this contingent far exceeded the total workforce of the Ministry of Health at the time (2.2 million health professionals).[25] In 1985, the Ministry of Health decided to stop using the name of barefoot doctors because of the large number of doctors, poor quality of their service, and the lack of standards in their training, use and assessment. Barefoot doctors passing examinations would be recognized as village doctors, while those failing to pass would become health workers.

Before the 1980s, China launched large-scale training of rural medical workers, creating a large contingent of medical workers serving the countryside. The training of barefoot doctors at the time had its unique characteristics, which were different from the traditional model in which Western medicine assumed dominance. Specifically, the training of barefoot doctors focused on the prevention and treatment of common diseases, frequently-occurring diseases, infectious diseases and endemic diseases in rural areas, and great importance was attached to ideological and political education (*i.e.* medical ethics education); since services based on Western medicine were expensive and would require medical equipment, which rural clinics could not afford, TCM knowledge and treatment methods, acupuncture in particular, were widely disseminated to barefoot doctors, and trainees were taught how to collect, grow, and make Chinese herbal medicines according to the local resources. In terms of teaching staff, there were members of mobile medical teams from Beijing or provincial capitals, medical personnel of regional hospitals, and doctors from county hospitals and commune health centers, but most of them were doctors from county hospitals and commune health centers because they

24 Department of Community-level Healthcare and MCH, Ministry of Health, ed. *Collection of Documents on Rural Healthcare (1951–2000)*. 302–304.

25 Zhang Kaining, ed. 2002. *From Barefoot Doctors to Village Doctors*. Kunming: Yunnan People's Publishing House. 20.

had a lot of practical experience in rural healthcare. This made the training efforts well-targeted at the needs of rural residents. In addition, the duration of training was not long, and initial training sessions were combined with follow-up training activities so that barefoot doctors kept improving themselves in practice. In short, under the cooperative medical care system, a set of large-scale, well-planned, independent and effective training mechanisms for rural barefoot doctors were gradually formed.

4 Significance of Rural Medical Practitioners' Training Model

Under a training model with Chinese characteristics, many rural medical workers were trained in a short period of time, which effectively alleviated the long-standing shortage of medical services and medicines and greatly improved the health of rural residents. The experience is still of relevance and significance to the development of the new countryside and the reform of China's healthcare system today.

First, such a training model suited China's national conditions and was the most feasible choice at the time. China's rural areas were vast, had a large population, and were uneven in terms of economic development. During the early years of the PRC, the country faced the poor health of residents and underdeveloped healthcare services. It was necessary to find a cost-effective model to train rural medical workers to meet the urgent need of disease prevention and treatment in rural areas, making up for the country's flaw in achieving nationwide coverage of healthcare services. The above-mentioned training model broke through the constraints of space and population and enabled the coverage of basic healthcare services in rural China to the largest extent. It offered the possibility of delivering primary healthcare in rural areas.

Second, such a training model produced medical workers who were able to stay in rural areas and serve rural residents. At the time, most of primary-level medical workers were selected from village communities, and when they returned to the communities they would serve their relatives, friends and fellow villagers. Such close relations made them more responsible when providing medical services and get along with the patients. In addition, they knew clearly where they could put their talent into use so they would stay in rural areas.

Third, such a model reduced training costs considerably. Since rural medical workers were all trained locally for a short period, and there would be follow-up training activities. They could keep improving themselves in practice and the training costs were greatly reduced. For that, barefoot doctors were produced at a low cost and were easy to support, which could be afforded by rural communities. The pay of barefoot doctors was only slightly higher than that of the general workforce (equivalent to the pay of production brigade officials at most), which was affordable for the cooperative medical care system. Besides, money was not paid in cash but in the form of year-end grain rations and wages like commune members. All these suited the realities of rural societies.

Fourth, such a training model connected rural medical care with its urban counterpart. The rural medical workers developed a closer relationship with the medical personnel of provincial, municipal, county and commune medical institutions. They introduced modern medicine, which had been widely applied in big cities to the countryside. Chen Zhiqian, hailed as "the father of China's public health" in academic circles, has a deep understanding of this point. As he said, community-based doctors are much needed. Much experience has shown that a health service system composed of dedicated administrators and even those at the village level with little training can indeed bring the benefits of medical knowledge to the villagers.[26]

Fifth, such a model was a great innovation in the national health system and provided a solid organizational system for the healthcare of rural residents. The system is based on the idea that in a country if it is impossible to ensure that there are senior doctors in every town or village. It is possible to ensure there is one or more middle-level health workers within walking distance for the majority of the population groups and even in many poor and remote areas. This model only adds the healthcare system to the existing political, economic, and administrative organizations. Many foreigners have spoken highly of this model. Assistant Director-General of the WHO Dr. Tadhada said that he had seen very few real primary healthcare like what China had and China's experience was of relevance to other developing countries since it had been proved to be truly effective. Professor Joao Tenney, President of the International Society of Rural Medicine, commented that China had made outstanding achievements in promoting public health and implementing primary healthcare, and set an example for other developing countries and that China's experience was useful not only to other developing countries but also to developed countries.[27]

Finally, this was markedly different from the Western model of medical care. First of all, in a complete overhaul of the traditional training in Western

26 C. C. Chen. 1998. *Medicine in Rural China: A Personal Account*. Chengdu: Sichuan People's Publishing House. 6–7.

27 Zhang Zikuan. 1994. "Drawing Upon Mao Zedong's Views on Healthcare." *Chinese Primary Health Care* 1.

medicine, setting the eligibility requirements for rural medical workers relatively low and offering the training to a large number of people helped to mitigate the tendency toward over-specialization in the practice of medicine. Traditional training in Western medicine had often been denied those who needed little more than relatively simple skills necessary for providing the most basics of medical care, such as treating common diseases, due in part to the belief that the integrity of Western medicine as a rarefied profession would otherwise be compromised. The Chinese model rejected this form of discrimination. Secondly, medical practitioners trained under this model mostly had similar socioeconomic background to those they treated. They were far more likely than doctors with superlative skills but not from the local area to be willing to devote their lives to the cause of serving people of the same social status as themselves. Moreover, that these locally trained doctors continued to work as farmers part-time effectively prevented a dichotomy from forming between the manual and the intellectual aspects of medical care. In sharp contrast with Western medicine, this model did not produce a group of elite physicians who had little in common with, and indeed occupied higher rungs on the social ladder than the masses they treated. Thirdly, barefoot doctors lived in the same environment as farmers, so they had a clear idea of patients' conditions. Fourthly, the rural medical workers trained in large number over a short period of time could satisfy the urgent needs of rural areas for healthcare. The development of barefoot doctors not only increased the accessibility of medical services but also promoted the dissemination of health-related knowledge, making the delivery of medical services not the exclusive right of medical professionals.

Overall, China gave full play to the creativity of the people, trained a large number of rural medical workers in a relatively short period of time, and managed to maximize the advantages of rich human resources and minimize the reliance on expensive medical technology or highly skilled medical personnel. The effect of this policy made it possible for China to face the challenge posed by the severe shortage of rural medical professionals. It also shows the great ambition of the country to creatively transform the medical care system for rural residents. As Joseph R. Levenson noted, the goal was not to find a Western model for China, but to build a Chinese model for the country that the West had long exploited and they wanted the key to solve their own problems from here (Chinese history).[28]

28 Joseph R. Levenson. 2000. *Confucian China and Its Modern Fate* (trans: Zheng Dahua and Ren Jing). Beijing: China Social Sciences Press. 316.

CHAPTER 14

Rural Cooperative Medical System in Historical Perspective

*Xia Xingzhen**

Abstract

Rural cooperative medical care is a collective healthcare system established by farmers in the People's Republic of China based voluntary mutual aid. It emerged when the agricultural cooperative movement was rising in the mid-1950s and developed quickly following the directives issued by Mao Zedong in January 1965 and on June 26, 1965. The discussions initiated by *The People's Daily* in 1968–1969 led to an upsurge in the number of medical cooperatives. After the Cultural Revolution, the cooperative medical scheme was gradually institutionalized. However, the number of traditional healthcare cooperatives has been shrinking since the 1980s. Since the 1990s, the CPC and the government have made great efforts to build a new cooperative medical scheme and a medical assistance system and continuously improve them. The country has accumulated a wealth of experience in managing rural cooperative medical care. As a practical model that suits China's national conditions, it effectively protects and promotes the health of farmers and is thus widely welcomed. The World Health Organization has also praised it.

Keywords

rural areas – cooperative medical care – barefoot doctors

More than 80 per cent of the Chinese populations live in rural areas. Due to the influence of many factors, such as social structure, geography, economy, living conditions and customs, rural areas lag far behind cities in access to sanitation and medical services and the overall well-being of residents. In 1945, Mao Zedong pointed out that "Public health is just empty talk if we leave out the

* Xia Xingzhen, research fellow at Contemporary China Institute.

 | DOI:10.1163/9789004737990_015

360 million rural population."[1] After the founding of the People's Republic of China, the CPC and the government attached great importance to the improvement in rural health. The PRC's first healthcare policy was geared towards the needs of workers, peasants and soldiers. The primary goal of developing healthcare was to improve access to healthcare in rural communities.[2] After years of hard work, remarkable progress was made. By the mid-1960s, the vast majority of counties, townships/communes, and villages/production team had built healthcare facilities, forming a basic rural healthcare network. However, the prolonged lack of healthcare resources in the vast rural areas was not fundamentally changed. Due to various reasons, the focus of health departments was still on cities. In 1964, 69 per cent of high-level health practitioners were in cities and 31 percent in rural areas (counties or lower-level administrative divisions), of which only 10 per cent were in rural areas below the county level. Of the country's intermediate health practitioners, 57 per cent were working in cities and 43 per cent in rural areas, of which only 27 per cent were in areas below the county level. TCM practitioners, on the contrary, mostly concentrated in rural areas. Cities accounted for 30 per cent of the government's total healthcare spending and the countryside accounted for 27 percent, of which only 16 percent was spent in areas below the county level. This means that the government spent more on the 8.3 million beneficiaries of the publicly funded health care scheme than on the 500 million farmers.[3] On June 26, 1965, Mao Zedong lambasted healthcare departments for this, and instructed them to "direct healthcare resources toward the countryside."[4] This prompted governments at all levels to attach importance to rural health, laying the foundation for the promotion of the rural cooperative medical model that emerged in the mid-1950s.

Cooperative medical care is a great initiative introduced by the farmers of the PRC in their long-term efforts to protect themselves from diseases, and has left its mark in the PRC's history of healthcare. It provides a solution to a common problem faced by all countries, especially developing countries. It is not only welcomed by Chinese farmers at home but also praised internationally.

1 Mao Zedong. 1991. *Selected Works of Mao Zedong* (*Vol. 3*). People's Publishing House. 1078.

2 Editorial Office of *Series on Contemporary China*, ed. 1986. *Healthcare in Contemporary China* (*Volume 2*). China Social Sciences Press. 43.

3 Report of the Party Committee of the Ministry of Health on the Task of Directing Healthcare Resources Toward the Countryside (submitted to Mao Zedong and the CCP Central Committee on August 11, 1965). In Department of Primary Care and Maternal and Child Health of the Ministry of Health (Ed.), *Collection of Rural Health Documents* (*1951–2000*) (p. 27). Printed in December 2001.

4 Mao Zedong. 1996. *Manuscripts by Mao Zedong after the Founding of the People's Republic* (*Volume 11*). Central Party Literature Press. 387.

At the 27th World Health Assembly in May 1974, representatives of developing countries showed strong interest in this model. The United Nation Women's and Children's Fund pointed out in its 1980–1981 annual report that China's barefoot doctors program provided primary care in backward rural areas and showed developing countries a way to improve access to healthcare.[5] The rural cooperative medical care model was hailed by the World Bank and the World Health Organization as the only effective healthcare funding model for developing countries.[6]

1 History of the Rural Cooperative Medical Care Scheme

1.1 *Cooperative Medical Care Emerged as Part of the Agricultural Cooperative Movement*

During the "Cultural Revolution", both cooperative medical care and barefoot doctors were promoted as "new initiatives" emerging in the health revolution. However, the fact is they appeared as early as the mid-1950s.[7]

"The cooperative medical system has gradually developed with the rise of the agricultural mutual aid and cooperative movement."[8] At that time, public officials and residents in some rural areas began to explore a mutual aid approach to healthcare. Commune members and collectives raised a certain amount of funds, and the production team paid members' medical expenses or a certain percentage thereof; the production team paid compensation to medical workers based on their work points. Generally speaking, the compensation of medical workers in rural areas was on the same level as middle-level laborers. When not treating patients, medical workers participated in agricultural production. During busy farming seasons, they would go to the field to provide medical services to farmers. For example, in 1957, the high-level agricultural production cooperative in Yangwu Township, Dongguan County, Guangdong Province, built a healthcare facility to treat minor injuries and illnesses for members of the cooperative and train barefoot doctors. After the commune

5 Health Research Institute of Kunming Medical College, ed. 2002. *From Barefoot Doctors to Rural Doctors*. Yunnan People's Publishing House, p. 5.

6 How Did Rural Areas in Jiangsu Handle SARS. *The People's Daily*, May 19, 2003.

7 The first appearance of "cooperative medical care" in the press was in January 1959. An article titled "Cooperative Medical Care in Cisheng People's Commune in Zhecheng County" was published in the first issue of the magazine *People's Health* in 1959. It reported that the Cisheng People's Commune in Zhecheng County, Henan Province began to adopt the cooperative medical care model on July 1, 1958.

8 Editorial Office of *Series on Contemporary China*, ed. 1986. *Healthcare in Contemporary China* (*Volume 2*). China Social Sciences Press. 65.

movement in 1958, a commune was responsible for paying for medical care provided to members. Later, after realizing that it was difficult to cover all the medical expenses as the collective economy was still weak, Yangwu Township decided to adopt the cooperative medical care model. Each member paid a fee of 0.15 yuan a month. Members paid the medical consultation fee out of pocket. The cooperative medical care scheme covered 70 percent of outpatient treatment costs and all hospitalization costs.[9]

1.2 *Mao Zedong's June 26 Directive Contributed to the Development of Cooperative Medical Care*

Cooperative medical care was designed with the situation of China's countryside in mind. It effectively improved access to healthcare in rural communities. Therefore, it was welcomed by rural residents and developed rapidly. In 1958, all 96 communes in Macheng County, Hubei Province, adopted the cooperative medical care model.[10] The National Rural Healthcare Conference held in Jishan County, Shanxi Province in November 1959 implemented this medical system, effectively driving the development of cooperative medical care. During the socialist education movement in rural areas, Mao Zedong gave a directive in January 1965, demanding health departments send urban high-level medical workers to rural areas to serve rural residents and train doctors for rural areas. On June 26, 1965, Mao Zedong instructed the Ministry of Health to direct healthcare resources toward the countryside (known as the "June 26 Directive"). These two important directives propelled health departments to attach more importance to rural health, and played an important role in promoting the cooperative medical model on a national scale and improving the skills of barefoot doctors. By the end of 1965, some counties in more than ten provinces, municipalities, and autonomous regions, including Shanxi, Hubei, Jiangxi, Jiangsu, Fujian, Guangdong, and Xinjiang, had adopted this model.[11]

1.3 *The Discussions Initiated by* The People's Daily *in 1968–1969 Led to an Upsurge in the Number of Large Healthcare Cooperatives*

The front cover of *The People's Daily* on December 5, 1968 has the headline, "Cooperative medical system is welcomed by poor and lower-middle peasants."

---

9 Cooperative Medical Care is Great – Investigation Report on Cooperative Medical Care in the Yangwu Production Team. *The People's Daily*, December 7, 1968.

10 Health Research Institute of Kunming Medical College, ed. 2002. *From Barefoot Doctors to Rural Doctors*. Yunnan People's Publishing House. 16.

11 Editorial Office of *Series on Contemporary China*, ed. 1986. *Healthcare in Contemporary China (Volume 2)*. China Social Sciences Press. 65.

This article reported on the experience of poor and lower-middle peasants in Leyuan Commune, Changyang County, Hubei Province in implementing the cooperative medical care model. This commune began to implement this model in December 1966. Every member paid a fee of 1 yuan per year to the medical cooperative and the production team paid 0.1 yuan for each participant from the public welfare fund. Except for a few chronic diseases, patients who had to take medicine all year round, members only needed to pay a medical consultation fee of 0.05 yuan each time they saw a doctor, and drugs were free. Of the 12 medical workers in the commune health center, except for 2 who received a fixed salary for the time being, the remaining 10 health workers were paid based on work points in the same way as the key officials of the production team. They also received a monthly subsidy ranging from 3 to 5 yuan. About 99 per cent of the people in the commune participated in the cooperative medical care scheme. The article summarizes the benefits of the cooperative medical care model. The most obvious one is improving access to healthcare in rural communities and protecting health of farmers. People often said, "Agricultural cooperatives rooted out poverty, and medical cooperatives rooted out disease."

From December 8, 1968 to December 4, 1969, *The People's Daily* initiated 23 rounds of discussions on the rural healthcare system, underlining the superiority of the cooperative medical system, sharing experiences in consolidating the system, and put forward suggestions for further improvement. Under the influence the discussions, rural medical cooperatives developed rapidly across the country in 1969.

From June 15 to 23, 1976, the National Barefoot Doctors Conference was held in Jiangzhen Commune, Chuansha County, Shanghai. After the meeting, the Ministry of Health submitted a report to the CPC Central Committee and the State Council on July 21, pointing out, "In areas where the barefoot doctors and cooperative medical care systems have been put in place, we must make full use of the two systems; in areas that have not yet adopted the two systems, especially border areas, communities of ethnic minorities, mountainous areas, old revolutionary bases, fishing areas, and pastoral areas, we should actively promote the two systems in a step-by-step manner and with local conditions in mind." By the end of 1977, 85 per cent of the production teams nationwide had adopted the cooperative medical care model.[12]

Rural communes implementing the cooperative medical care model had formed an effective management system. Take Leyuan Commune in

12 Department of Primary Care and Maternal and Child Health of the Ministry of Health, ed. 2001. *Collection of Rural Health Documents (1951–2000)*. 419.

Changyang County, Hubei Province, for example. The commune set up a cooperative medical care management committee, and the production team set up a management team accordingly. They were responsible for managing the cooperative medical care program under the leadership of the commune revolutionary committee and the leading group of the production team. They regularly reported to the public and listened to the opinions of the masses.[13]

Needless to say, influenced by extreme left politics during the "Cultural Revolution", some local governments did make some mistakes when implementing the cooperative medical models and catered to political needs too much. Such mistakes included unreasonable use of administrative orders, excessive ambition when it came to coverage, and over-reliance on "one-size-fits-all" policies that ignored differences in communes. These mistakes compromised this system. In addition, formalism had also hindered the development of the healthcare sector in some areas.

1.4 *After the End of the "Cultural Revolution", Rural Cooperative Medical Care Was Gradually Institutionalized*

After the end of the "Cultural Revolution", after getting rid of drawbacks brought about by politicization, the country adopted a more pragmatic approach to promote the rural cooperative medical care model. In order to keep the development of this model on the right track, the Ministry of Health worked with relevant departments to formulate national regulations and standards for the operation of the model. In December 1979, the Ministry of Health, the Ministry of Agriculture, the Ministry of Finance, the State Administration of Medicine, and the All-China Federation of Supply and Marketing Cooperatives jointly issued *Notice on Rural Cooperative Medical Care Regulations (Draft)*. It points out that the development of the rural cooperative medical care model played a positive role in improving access to healthcare in rural areas and protecting the health of commune members. It instructs local health departments to strengthen leadership, continue to sum up experience, and properly solve existing problems, so as to further improve the rural cooperative medical care model and support agricultural modernization. *Rural Cooperative Medical Care Regulations (Draft)* is the first official regulatory document issued by a government department. Its content includes general rules, goals, forms and management institutions of cooperative medical care, funds and management systems, barefoot doctors and hygienists, midwifery, Chinese herbal medicine,

13 Changyang County, Hubei Province,"We have focused on three major goals – the experience of the Yuetuan Commune in implementing the cooperative medical system". *The People's Daily*, December 11, 1968.

and strengthening leadership. It is a comprehensive and detailed policy on cooperative medical care. It summarizes the experience of rural cooperative medical care in the previous 20 years, and is a symbol of the institutionalisation of cooperative medical care.

In February 1981, the State Council approved and forwarded the Ministry of Health's *Report on Reasonably Solving the Problems Concerning Subsidies for Barefoot Doctors*. This document has also played a very important role in improving the cooperative medical care model. According to the report, barefoot doctors were important actors in healthcare and family planning in rural areas, and about one-third of them had completed secondary vocational education or had equivalent education experience. Like teachers of people-run schools, they were rural intellectuals and technicians. Compensation was a crucial issue in the development of barefoot doctors. *Report on Reasonably Solving the Problems Concerning Subsidies for Barefoot Doctors* suggests that "All barefoot doctors who have passed their qualifying exams and completed secondary vocational education or had equivalent education experience should be issued a rural doctor certificate and, in principle, be given compensation and benefits at the same level as teachers of local private schools." "At the same time, the commune or the production team should give them work points." For barefoot doctors who had not completed secondary vocational education or had no equivalent education experience, the commune or the production team should "provide them with a subsidy in addition to compensation based on work points when conditions permit." The report also points out that "the county health bureau should be responsible for the transfer, training, assessment, and certification of barefoot doctors and operation of barefoot doctor subsidy schemes." These policies and regulations played an important role in promoting the development of barefoot doctors and improving the cooperative medical model. In 1980, about 90 per cent of the administrative villages (production teams) in China implemented cooperative medical care, and healthcare schemes covered 85 per cent of the rural population.[14]

1.5 *In the 1980s, Rural Cooperative Medical Care Began to Decline*

From the late 1970s to the mid-1980s, China's rural economy underwent tremendous changes. With the introduction of the household responsibility system and the abolition of the people's commune system, new rural economic and administrative systems gradually took shape. Rural primary care facilities and the cooperative medical care model were also overhauled.

14 Department of Primary Care and Maternal and Child Health of the Ministry of Health, ed. 2001. *Collection of Rural Health Documents (1951–2000)*. 533–534.

For a considerable period of time, rural cooperative medical care showed a declining trend. The main reasons are: (1) Rural cooperative medical care was a socialist welfare scheme. In the initial stage of the rural economic reform, many local governments found increasing the funding for welfare programs difficult. Many areas saw a drop in welfare funding. The lack of welfare funding seriously affected the development of cooperative medical care; (2) The number of medical workers was decreasing. On the one hand, the relaxing of rural policies led to increased ways to make money. Some rural medical workers gave up their career to work in other industries. On the other hand, barefoot doctors emerged and rose in parallel with cooperative medical care, and the name, practices, and service nature of barefoot doctors were no longer compatible with the new conditions that emerged after the reform and opening up. According to the *Report on Reasonably Solving the Problems Concerning Subsidies for Barefoot Doctors* approved by the State Council in 1981, 1.25 million barefoot doctors were assessed, and 640,000 received the rural doctor certificate. The Ministry of Health decided in 1985 to stop using the term "barefoot doctor".[15] As a result, the number of rural medical workers dropped by 50 per cent, and no new medical workers came to rural areas. Of course, cooperative medical care was affected.

Due to the reasons mentioned above, cooperative medical care was declining fast. At the end of the 1980s, the participation rate of cooperative medical care dropped to 4.8 per cent. Cooperative medical care programs were shut down. Most farmers could not afford medical care, and many of them fell into or returned to poverty due to disease.

1.6 *In the 1990s, China Began to Step Up Efforts to Improve the Cooperative Medical Model*

The CPC and the Chinese government tried very hard to reverse the decline of rural cooperative medical care.

On January 17, 1991, the State Council approved *the Request for Heath Reform That Increases Rural Medical and Health Workers* submitted by the Ministry of Health and other departments, which proposed to "steadily promote the cooperative medical care model and support efforts that expand comprehensive coverage and access for all citizens in China."[16] This report affirmed the merits of the cooperative medical care model, summed up past experience, and

15 Health Research Institute of Kunming Medical College, ed. 2002. *From Barefoot Doctors to Rural Doctors*. Yunnan People's Publishing House. 22.

16 Department of Primary Care and Maternal and Child Health of the Ministry of Health, ed. 2001. *Collection of Rural Health Documents (1951–2000)*. 84–85, 105.

proposed measures to improve the cooperative medical care model in the future. Rural cooperative medical care was a constant subject in the government documents on rural health issued subsequently.

In 1994, the Ministry of Health and other departments of the Chinese government cooperated with the World Health Organization to launch a Study of Rural Cooperative Medical Care Reform in China. An international conference was held in Shanghai in early July to officially announce the project's launch.[17]

The National Healthcare Conference held in December 1996 put the restoration, development and improvement of rural cooperative medical care on its agenda. Jiang Zemin pointed out at the conference, "In poverty-stricken areas, poverty alleviation should be combined with healthcare. Nowadays, many rural areas have won people's hearts by implementing the cooperative medical care model. People call cooperative medical care "heart-winning" or "moral governance project". The key to improving access to healthcare in rural communities is to develop and improve cooperative medical care. This is an observation made based on past experience over a long period. It is in line with China's national conditions and farmers' wishes. We should achieve a further consensus on this issue, strengthen leadership, and prudently handle relevant matters." Li Peng said at the conference, "We have made it clear that the three-level (county, township, and village levels) health service network, cooperative medical care, and rural doctors are the three pillars of rural health. This direction is correct, and we must earnestly stick to it." He also said, "Rural cooperative medical care is a basic rural healthcare system with Chinese characteristics. It is a major issue related to party-mass relations, rural economic development, and social stability. We must handle it well and deepen health reforms to support the sustainable development of cooperative medical care."

Decision of the CPC Central Committee on Several Issues Concerning the Establishment of a Socialist Market Economic System and *Outline of the Ninth Five-Year Plan on National Economic and Social Development and Long-Term Goal for 2010* approved by the Fourth Session of the Eighth National People's Congress emphasized the necessity to develop and improve various forms of rural cooperative medical care with local reality in mind. *Decision of the CPC Central Committee and the State Council on Health Reform and Development* points out, "Cooperative medical care plays an important role in ensuring farmers' access to basic medical services, achieving preventive healthcare targets, and preventing poverty caused by illness ... We should ensure that most rural areas

17 Documents of the Ministry of Health.

have adopted various cooperative medical care programs by 2000 and gradually increased social support for healthcare."[18]

To implement the above-mentioned decisions of the CPC Central Committee, the National People's Congress, and the State Council, several ministries, including the Ministry of Health and the State Planning Commission, the Ministry of Finance, the Ministry of Agriculture, and the Ministry of Civil Affairs, jointly submitted *Opinions on the Development and Improvement of Rural Cooperative Medical Care* to the State Council. On May 28, 1997, this document was approved and released by the State Council. To involve all stakeholders, the Ministry of Health issued *Notice on Further Promoting Cooperative Medical Care* on November 7, 1997. The Notice requires relevant departments to: (i) carry out comprehensive publicity activities to make citizens aware of the merits of cooperative medical care; (ii) improve the management, efficiency, service delivery, and supervision of cooperative medical care, ensure cooperative medical care programs truly benefit citizens, and underscore that scientific management is the key to sustainable development of cooperative medical care; (iii) strengthen training of medical workers, which is the basis for the start and development of cooperative medical care programs; and (iv) make full use of exemplary models, which is an effective way to promote the development and improvement of cooperative medical care. The Annual Report on Rural Cooperative Medical Care appended to the notice requires county-level health departments that launched a cooperative medical care program to report to the provincial health departments.

1.7 *At the Beginning of the 21st Century, the Chinese Government Proposed to Establish New Rural Cooperative Medical Care and Medical Assistance Systems and Continuously Improve Them*

To establish a rural health system that corresponds to the socialist market economy suits economic and social conditions in China's rural areas, and has preventive and basic medical functions, the State Council Office for Restructuring the Economic System, the State Planning Commission, the Ministry of Finance, the Ministry of Agriculture, and the Ministry of Health jointly proposed *Guidelines for Rural Health Reform and Development*, which was forwarded by the General Office of the State Council on May 24, 2001. The document requires that local people's governments at all levels strengthen the organisation and leadership of cooperative medical care, continue to improve cooperative medical care with local reality in mind. Citizens should participate in cooperative

18 Department of Primary Care and Maternal and Child Health of the Ministry of Health, ed. 2001. *Collection of Rural Health Documents (1951–2000)*. 125.

medical care programs voluntarily. The private sector should play a major role in cooperative medical care, and the government should provide support. Members should be the main source of funds for cooperative medical care. Collectives and the government should provide the necessary financial support. Financial transparency and democratic management must be ensured. In areas where conditions permit, it is recommended that counties (cities) plan for serious illness and help farmers reduce the burden of the exorbitant costs of treating critical illnesses, which most individuals and families cannot afford. In October 2002, the CPC Central Committee and the State Council issued *Decision on Further Improving Rural Healthcare*, setting out regulations and measures for the rural cooperative medical care reform and pointing out that "governments at all levels should increase health investment year by year, and the growth rate should not be less than the growth rate of fiscal expenditures over the same period." On October 30, Li Lanqing proposed in his speech at the National Rural Healthcare Conference that the country should build new rural cooperative medical care and medical assistance systems, which could effectively help farmers reduce the burden of the exorbitant costs of treating critical illnesses. This new medical care system is essentially a mutual aid and cooperation system for farmers, guided and supported by the government. It focuses on helping farmers pay medical and hospitalization expenses that they could not afford. Beginning in 2003, counties were selected to run pilot projects as part of the country's effort to accumulate practical experience and promote the new rural cooperative medical care system in a step-by-step manner. By 2010, almost all rural areas across the country had launched rural healthcare and rural cooperative medical care schemes that corresponded to the socialist market economy and suited economic and social conditions in the countryside.

On August 8, 2003, Beijing held a rural healthcare conference and put forward specific measures to promote the development of the new cooperative medical system. The Beijing city announced that the municipal government would invest 200 million yuan within three years to improve rural healthcare and launch critical illness insurance for rural residents. Since that year, financial departments of at municipal, district, county, and township levels have begun to provide fixed subsidies for areas that offered critical illness insurance to farmers. Among them, the municipal financial department of Beijing planned to pay 50 million yuan in the form of subsidy to participants of the cooperative medical care scheme each year, including 10 yuan per participant living in suburban areas, 5 yuan per participant in plain areas in suburban counties, and 20 yuan per participant in mountainous areas. [9] In addition to Beijing, other cities actively explored new rural cooperative medical care models.

2 China's Experiences in Implementing the Rural Cooperative Medical Care Model

Since the rise of rural cooperative medical care in the mid-1950s, China has implemented the model for nearly 50 years. This system with Chinese characteristics has experienced many twists and turns, resulting in a wealth of experiences and lessons. The following is a summary of what we have learned.

2.1 *Achieving Consensus and Strengthening Leadership Are the Keys to Developing and Improving Rural Cooperative Medical Care*

The rural cooperative medical care system is suitable for China's conditions. It can effectively meet the needs of farmers, who account for most of the Chinese population, and safeguard their health. To improve rural healthcare, the key is improving the cooperative medical care system. The cooperative medical care model seeks fundamental benefits for farmers and meets their two needs for health and well-being. It is a practical tool for good governance and has won the broad support of farmers. The model guarantees the quality of the rural labour force and the stability and harmony of rural families, thereby effectively increasing agricultural productivity and maintaining the stability of rural society. It drives the economic and social development of socialist China and contributes to the country's prosperity. Previous CPC leaders, including Mao Zedong, Deng Xiaoping, and Jiang Zemin, all attached great importance to and vigorously advocated this model., Leaders at all levels have recognised the necessity and merits of cooperative medical care from the central to grassroots level. Helping farmers solve challenges and problems encountered in implementing this model and in the process of deepening reforms is the key to the consolidation, improvement and development of rural cooperative medical care. I believe that the superiority of socialism with Chinese characteristics will be vividly demonstrated by improving this unique model.

2.2 *The Private Sector Should Be the Primary Source of Funds and the Government Should Provide Necessary Support. Scientific Management That Suits Local Conditions Should Be Ensured*

Cooperative medical care is a social welfare undertaking based on mutual assistance and cooperation. Its funds mainly come from two sources. One is the contribution of farmers and rural families, and the other is the contribution of collectives at all levels. In October 2002, the CPC Central Committee and the State Council issued *a Decision to Further Improve Rural Health*, stipulating that individual farmers, the local financial department and the state should each contribute 10 yuan to the cooperative medical care scheme. Since then, the state has become one of the three sources of funds for cooperative medical care, and the funding of the cooperative medical care scheme has been met. Where conditions permit, financial departments at both township and village levels support the scheme financially. Therefore, the development of collective economic activities at township and village levels is the key to the scheme's consolidation, development and improvement.

The management of cooperative medical care should be based on the actual conditions of each administrative division. Over-reliance on the one-size-fits-all approach is unacceptable.

2.3 *Barefoot Doctors and Itinerant Health Workers Were the Backbone of Rural Cooperative Medical Care, and the Country Must Promote the Development of Barefoot Doctors and Itinerant Health Workers Based on the Actual Situation*

Due to limited funding, training affordable doctors is crucial for cooperative medical care. This is where barefoot doctors who did not receive wages or leave the production team could come into play. They were one of the key actors in cooperative medical care. Who was responsible for training barefoot doctors? In addition to hospitals at county and commune/township levels, the itinerant medical teams built following the directives issued by Mao Zedong in January 1965, and on June 26, 1965 were sent by urban and military hospitals to the countryside to train barefoot doctors. It should be noted that barefoot doctors and itinerant health workers played an essential role in developing cooperative medical care.

Barefoot doctors were coined by poor and lower-middle peasants in the suburbs of Shanghai to refer to hygienists who participated in agricultural activities and provided medical services simultaneously. This term first appeared in a report entitled "Forecasting the direction of the medical education revolution based on the growth of barefoot doctors – a survey report of Shanghai City" in the third issue of the year 1968 of *Red Flag* published on September 10, 1968. Because the term vividly described the characteristics of this group, it was quickly accepted by the general public. The rapid development of barefoot doctors contributed to establishing the rural cooperative medical system.

Barefoot doctors and cooperative medical care were complementary. In the early days of cooperative medical care, only communes had medical workers who rarely visited production teams. It was inconvenient for farmers to see a doctor. Health departments at all levels began to increase efforts to cultivate grassroots health workers. They selected persons with proper political awareness and good moral character from production brigades and production teams. They trained them after obtaining approval from the commune's cooperative medical care management committee. These farmers participated in training when they were not busy with farm work. They would return to production teams during busy farm months. In April 1964, the Department of Medical Education of the Ministry of Health issued *Opinions on Continuing to Strengthen the Training of Health Workers and Midwives in Rural Areas Without Leaving Production Teams* (*Draft for Comments*) and distributed copies of the document to health departments or bureaus of provinces, cities, and autonomous regions and 41 medical colleges and universities. The document proposes that "from 1965, within 3 to 5 years, we will strive to ensure that every production brigade has a midwife and every production team has a hygienist." "They will mainly be engaged in agricultural production. At the same time, they will also provide medical services to the masses."[19] This document provided guidance for the training and development of barefoot doctors.

The number of barefoot doctors in China reached the highest in the 1970s. There were more than 1.5 million of them and more than 3.9 million hygienists and birth attendants in production teams at the time. More than 5 million people were engaged in healthcare in rural areas,[20]which was more than twice the total number of health workers (2.2 million) under the Ministry of Health. Cooperative medical care provided barefoot doctors with opportunities to practice medicine and become qualified doctors; barefoot doctors were the main actors in the delivery of cooperative medical care. They played a crucial role in rural healthcare and the protection of the health of farmers. Some rightly commented, "Cooperative medical care is mainly done through barefoot doctors."[21]

Itinerant medical teams play a supportive role in developing cooperative medical care. After the founding of the People's Republic of China, itinerant medical teams were built to provide services to rural areas and communities of ethnic minorities. In January 1965, Mao Zedong instructed high-level medical workers in urban areas to go to the countryside to train doctors for rural communities. The Party Group of the Ministry of Health immediately discussed this matter and invited some representatives from the National People's Congress and the CPPCC to participate in the discussion. On January 19 and 20, the Party Group of the Ministry of Health submitted a report on implementing the

19 Health Research Institute of Kunming Medical College, ed. 2002. *From Barefoot Doctors to Rural Doctors*. Yunnan People's Publishing House. 17.

20 Data on barefoot doctors, production team hygienists, and birth attendants are from Department of Primary Care and Maternal and Child Health of the Ministry of Health, ed. 2001. *Collection of Rural Health Documents (1951–2000)*. 420.

21 Health Research Institute of Kunming Medical College, ed. 2002. *From Barefoot Doctors to Rural Doctors*. Yunnan People's Publishing House. 315.

above instruction to the CPC Central Committee and Chairman Mao Zedong. This report summarises this report: (1) The Ministry of Health planned to send high-level medical teams to rural areas in batches to train grassroots health workers. They would first visit key counties for social education to support the Four Clean-ups Movement and offer medical workers guidance on ethical conduct and practices. This itinerant arrangement would become a long-term mechanism in the future. Beijing was selecting the first batch of itinerant medical workers who would go to the countryside after the Spring Festival. (2) The Ministry of Health also planned to continue to improve medical education. Many medical schools would shorten school terms and increase enrollment. Many qualified intermediate medical schools would set up specialties. TCM schools would shorten school terms, improve their specialty programs' teaching policies and job assignments, and train medical workers for rural areas. They would continue to strengthen the training of medical workers who would continue to be part of agricultural production teams in rural areas. These medical workers would treat minor injuries and diseases, assist in childbirth, and be part of mass health campaigns. Mao Zedong approved this report on January 21.[22] On January 31, the Ministry of Health issued a *Notice on Issues Related to Itinerant Medical Workers for Rural Areas* and made arrangements timely. On February 6, 1965, the CPC Central Committee publicly announced Chairman Mao Zedong's instructions and the Ministry of Health's report, pointing out that "this is a path the healthcare sector must take. It focuses on serving workers, peasants and soldiers. Health departments should sum up experiences promptly."[23]

Beijing and other major cities across the country quickly built itinerant medical teams and sent them to rural areas, mountainous areas, pastoral areas, and forest areas to serve local people following Mao Zedong's instructions. According to estimation, as of mid-April 1965, 1,521 medical teams were built nationwide, and 18,697 medical workers (including those of county hospitals) participated in the itinerant medical worker program. In the first half of 1965, cities sent more than 28,000 medical workers to the countryside.[24] The itinerant medical teams built by most provinces and autonomous regions had first-class experts, professors, and famous TCM practitioners.

22 Mao Zedong. 1996. *Manuscripts by Mao Zedong after the Founding of the People's Republic (Volume 11)*. Central Party Literature Press. 318.

23 Health Research Institute of Kunming Medical College, ed. 2002. *From Barefoot Doctors to Rural Doctors*. Yunnan People's Publishing House. 625.

24 Including about 17,000 medical workers of county hospitals. Data are from the General Office of the Ministry of Health, ed. The 1st and 2nd Issues of *Briefings of Itinerant Medical Teams*, April 17,1965 and April 24, 1965.

Itinerant medical teams did their work, including performing operations, under challenging conditions. They helped cure many common diseases effectively and efficiently, saved the lives of many critically ill patients, and made many blind people see again. Therefore, local residents welcomed itinerant medical teams. In addition to providing medical care, another responsibility of itinerant medical teams was training medical workers for rural communities. Local people praised them for leaving behind medical teams that would not leave. This itinerant medical worker program was later institutionalized. In the 1960s and 1970s, thousands of people from the Beijing medical team visited Gansu, Shaanxi, Yunnan, Jiangxi and other provinces and Ali Prefecture of Tibet to provide medical care to people of all ethnic groups. Shanghai, Liaoning, Jiangsu, Shandong, Henan, Hunan, Hubei, Sichuan and other provinces and municipalities also sent medical teams to Tibet. The People's Liberation Army sent many medical workers to support rural areas. All provinces, municipalities, and autonomous regions sent medical workers to remote rural areas within their jurisdiction. By 1975, cities and the People's Liberation Army had sent more than 1.1 million medical workers to rural area, bringing health knowledge and medical services to the countryside. They played an important role in improving access to healthcare in rural communities and promoting rural health development, including the rural cooperative medical care model.

Training and practice had allowed barefoot doctors to improve their medical knowledge and skills continuously. In October 1974, when Deng Xiaoping met with a health delegation from another developing country, he affirmed the barefoot doctor model. He said barefoot doctors were no longer barefooted and, in fact they were wearing straw sandals or even cloth shoes. It was a metaphor for barefoot doctors' improved medical knowledge and skills.[25] Later, the barefoot doctors model completed its historical mission. Those who passed the qualification examination were awarded the village doctor certificate. This marked the further institutionalization of the cooperative medical care model and improved rural medical care. This itinerant medical worker model was also developed. Large hospitals and TCM hospitals in cities were required to provide targeted assistance, itinerant medical workers, and train health workers for rural communities. In addition, urban doctors were required to serve in rural areas for one year before being promoted to attending physicians or deputy chief physicians.[26]

---

25 Health Research Institute of Kunming Medical College, ed. 2002. *From Barefoot Doctors to Rural Doctors*. Yunnan People's Publishing House. 22–23.

26 Decision of the CPC Central Committee and the State Council on Further Improving Rural Health. October 2002. Implications of SARS on China's Effort to Improve Rural Health. *Guangming Daily*, May 16, 2003.

2.4 *To Promote the Sustainable Development of Cooperative Medical Care, Health Departments Must Prioritize Preventive Care and Integrate Chinese and Western Medicine*

Prioritizing preventive care was one of the four major health policies in the early days of the PRC. Barefoot doctors actively worked with production teams to promote hygiene habits, help residents fight unsanitary habits, and launch a patriotic sanitation campaign centered on the elimination of pests and diseases. This nationwide sanitation campaign included actions to strengthen management of feces and drinking water sources and improve toilets, livestock pens, water wells, environment and stoves. The campaign greatly improved rural sanitation. Integration of Chinese and Western medicine is a major feature of rural healthcare in China. It has also contributed to the development of cooperative medical care. Mao Zedong once said, "Chinese medicine is a great treasure house. Efforts should be made to improve and make full use of it."[27] In the long-term struggle with diseases, Chinese farmers have accumulated extensive experience in using Chinese herbal medicine, acupuncture, cupping therapy and other TCM materials and therapies. TCM materials are cheap and easy to obtain and are welcomed by Chinese farmers. When promoting cooperative medical care, the CPC and the government advocated utilization of local medical resources. Some areas encouraged local people to start business by using local medicine and prescriptions. Many communes and brigades set up TCM factories. These methods effectively improved access to healthcare in rural communities and reduced the medical expenses of farmers and the expenditure of the cooperative medical care scheme.

Rural cooperative medical care was chosen by the CPC, the government and farmers based on the real conditions of the countryside, and the country at large. The CPC and the Chinese government attach great importance to learning from the practices concerning rural cooperative medical care in the past several decades, and supporting the system's restoration, reconstruction, development and improvement. The SARS outbreak in the spring and summer of 2003 made Chinese people more keenly realize the necessity of rural cooperative medical care, the important role of rural doctors in epidemic prevention, the advantages of TCM in steadily cooling down human temperatures, shortening the duration of symptoms, reducing the amount of hormones in severely ill patients, maintaining blood oxygen concentration, and reducing the impact of viruses on hematopoiesis.[28] It validated once again the

27 Mao Zedong. 1983. *Selected Works of Mao Zedong*. People's Publishing House. 545.

28 Li Jiajie. A Milestone in Promoting Traditional Chinese Medicine – The Role of China Academy of Chinese Medical Sciences in the Fight against SARS. *Guangming Daily*, July 10, 2003.

correctness of the policies of serving the countryside, prioritizing prevention, and integrating Chinese and Western medicine, which were established in the early days of the PRC. Chinese people have learned a lot from this fight against SARS. I believe that under the leadership of the CPC Central Committee led by General Secretary Hu Jintao, Chinese people will further improve the new rural cooperative medical care system and safeguard the health of the 900 million farmers in China.

CHAPTER 15

Prioritizing the Countryside in Healthcare Development

A Review of Mao Zedong's June 26 Directive

*Yao Li**

Abstract

In 1965, rural areas in China was facing a shortage of healthcare resources. At the time, the country was giving priority to the development of heavy industry. The Ministry of Health had long concentrated its human, material and financial resources in cities. To improve access to healthcare in rural communities, Mao Zedong instructed the Ministry of Health to direct healthcare resources toward the countryside (known as the "June 26 Directive"). This directive reflects Mao's commitment to the mass line, utter condemnation of bureaucracy, and his consideration of war preparedness. Implementing the June 26 Directive effectively promoted the development of cooperative healthcare and a model of rural healthcare delivery employing itinerant health workers, significantly improving access to healthcare in rural communities. This study of the June 26 Directive is practically significant because it can provide information for studies of current healthcare reforms and support evidence-based policymaking concerning the rural healthcare system.

Keywords

Mao Zedong – cooperative healthcare system – June 26 Directive

On June 26, 1965, following a conversation with his doctor, Mao Zedong instructed the Ministry of Health to direct healthcare resources toward the countryside to improve rural residents' access to healthcare resources and increase the provision of medical care to the large rural population (known as the "June 26 Directive"). The directive had an important impact on China's

* Yao Li, associate researcher at Contemporary China Institute.

 | DOI:10.1163/9789004737990_016

healthcare system, especially in rural areas. In recent years, as healthcare reforms continue to deepen and problems in the rural healthcare system become increasingly prominent, this directive has been frequently cited, either to showcase the achievement made by China in rural healthcare or to criticize the Chinese government's long-standing neglect of rural healthcare. In the face of mixed reviews and the current grim situation of rural healthcare, we must re-examine the ins and outs, cause and consequences of the June 26 Directive and draw lessons from the past.

1 Historic Context of the June 26 Directive

When the People's Republic of China was founded, health professionals faced a healthcare system riddled with defects. After 16 years of hard work, China's healthcare sector developed quickly, dramatically improving the health and well-being of Chinese people. Cholera was soon eliminated in the country. In 1955, China effectively controlled the bubonic plague. In 1959, sexually transmitted diseases were eliminated nationwide. Smallpox was successfully eradicated in China in the early 1960s, a dozen years earlier than the worldwide eradication. The death rate of tuberculosis dropped from 250 per 100,000 in the early days of the People's Republic of China to 40 per 100,000 in the early 1960s. The incidence of infectious diseases such as polio, leprosy, Japanese encephalitis, diphtheria, tetanus, and whooping cough dropped significantly. In 1965, the number of birth attendants rose to 685,740, and the incidence of puerperal fever and neonatal tetanus was reduced considerably. The country achieved significant gains in maternal and newborn health.[1] The three-level rural primary health network with communes at the center actively improved rural sanitation and protected rural residents' health. Despite such remarkable progress, Mao Zedong criticized the Ministry of Health for focusing on the urban population, which accounted for only 15 per cent of the country's total population, especially public officials, and neglecting the majority of farmers. The directive came as a shock to the healthcare sector because the country's healthcare policy established in the early days had been focusing on serving workers, peasants and soldiers, and they had made remarkable progress in rural healthcare.[2] Was the June 26 Directive a proper policy in light of the

1 Editorial Office of *Series on Contemporary China*, ed. 1986. *Healthcare in Contemporary China (Part 1)*. China Social Sciences Press. 10–13.

2 Zhang Zikuan. 2006. Review and Evaluation of the Historical Context of the June 26 Directive. *China Rural Health Management* (9).

historical context? What prompted Mao to criticise the Ministry of Health in such a harsh way? To answer these questions, we need to compare urban and rural healthcare systems at the time and analyze the shift of the healthcare focus 16 years after the founding of the People's Republic of China.

1.1 *A Wide Rural-Urban Gap in the Coverage of Healthcare Schemes*

Protecting and promoting public health has always been a mission of the Communist Party of China (CPC). Therefore, as soon as the PRC was founded, building a health insurance system was put on the agenda of the Chinese government. The healthcare schemes for employees of state-owned enterprises (SOEs) and for public officials were rolled out. Urban employees, public officials, teachers and college students only needed to pay medical consultation fees and house call fees out of pocket, and SOEs or the state paid other medical expenses. SOEs also paid 50 per cent of medical expenses for their employees' immediate family members. The publicly funded healthcare scheme for public officials also covered the medical expenses of the children of public officials. Given the country's economic conditions and the actual situation in rural areas at time, China couldn't expand these schemes to cover rural areas in the short term. Although the government had also provided a lot of support for rural communities, including free treatment of some infectious diseases and medical assistance to poor households, rural residents paid most of medical expenses out of pocket. After the rural cooperative movement in 1955, some farmers set up healthcare mutual aid cooperatives. In 1965, some counties in more than ten provinces, including Shaanxi, Hubei, Jiangsu, Guangdong, and Xinjiang, adopted this healthcare cooperative model, but the benefits were incomparable to those provided by urban healthcare schemes.

There was another problem in the urban healthcare system. A small number of people were manipulating the system funded by SOEs and the government, leading to an increase in the waste of healthcare resources. Therefore, the central government repeatedly proposed reforming the two schemes. In 1957, Zhou Enlai pointed out in *Report on Remunerations and Other Benefits* at the Third Plenary Session of the Eighth CPC Central Committee, "Due to the unreasonable system design and poor management, waste in the publicly funded healthcare system is extremely serious." Not only is there a huge waste of funds, but also a more incredible waste of human resources, medical equipment, and medicines.[3] He required improvements on the two schemes,

3 Party Literature Research Office of the CPC Central Committee, ed. 1994. *Collection of Major Government Documents of the People's Republic of China (Volume 10)*. Central Party Literature Press. 587.

asking for a small medical fee to be charged. This was the first time the central government mentioned the problems in the urban healthcare schemes in an official document and called for healthcare reform. After Mao issued the June 26 Directive, the central government reaffirmed the necessity to reform the two schemes.[4] In response to the central government's instructions, the Ministry of Health and the Ministry of Finance issued *Notice on Improving the Management of Publicly Funded Health Care*, making appropriate adjustments to the public official healthcare scheme and requiring all units to strengthen management and avoid overspending. On April 15, 1966, the Ministry of Labor and the All-China Federation of Trade Unions jointly issued a *Notice on Several Issues Concerning the Improvement of the SOE Employees' Healthcare Scheme*, proposing ways to improve the scheme. These policies reflected the determination of the central government to reduce the rural-urban gap in access to healthcare.

1.2 *Huge Rural-Urban Disparities in Distribution and Input of Healthcare Resources*

Before the founding of the People's Republic of China, most of the country's healthcare institutions and human resources were concentrated in cities and coastal areas. There were few rural healthcare facilities. Only a few traditional Chinese medicine (TCM) practitioners provided limited medical services to rural residents. The newly founded republic faced the immediate task of improving access to healthcare in rural areas. In 1950, Zhou Enlai announced the plan "to establish a healthcare agency in each county or district to promote public health."[5] By the end of 1952, 90 per cent of China's counties had established their health facilities. By 1965, the rural healthcare network was completed, with 880,000 practitioners, and it grew much faster than that of the cities.[6] Nevertheless, there was still a considerable rural-urban gap in access to healthcare resources.

After issuing the June 26 Directive, the Ministry of Health reviewed the mistakes they had made in the report submitted to Mao Zedong and the CPC Central Committee: "As the leaders of the Ministry of Health have concentrated human, material, and financial resources in cities for a prolonged period

4 The CCP Central Committee Approved and Forwarded the Report of the Party Committee of the Ministry of Health on the Task of Directing Healthcare Resources Toward the Countryside. In Department of Primary Care and Maternal and Child Health of the Ministry of Health, ed. *Collection of Rural Health Documents (1951–2000)* (p. 26).

5 Author unknown. *Selected Works of Zhou Enlai (Volume 2)*. 1984. People's Publishing House. 48.

6 National Bureau of Statistics. *China Statistical Yearbook (2003)*. 2003. China Statistics Press. 806.

of time, the problem of lack of healthcare resources in rural areas has not been resolved so far. In 1964, 69 per cent of high-level health practitioners were in cities and 31 per cent in rural areas, of which only 10 per cent were working below the county level. Not only was the number of health workers (including both TCM and Western medicine practitioners) on a per capita basis in rural areas much lower than that in cities, but the skills of most health workers in rural areas were also meagre. The Chinese government spent more than 930 million yuan in healthcare that year, of which more than 280 million yuan was spent on publicly funded healthcare in urban areas, accounting for 30 per cent of the government's total healthcare spending. More than 250 million yuan was spent in rural areas, accounting for 27 per cent, of which only 16 per cent was spent on healthcare below the county level. This means the government spent more on the 8.3 million beneficiaries of publicly funded healthcare schemes than the 500 million farmers.[7] These figures show a vast rural-urban gap in healthcare access at the time. The cause of the gap was very complicated, and the influence of the country's industrialisation goals was one of the major factors contributing to the gap.

In the early days of the People's Republic of China, given the shortage of healthcare resources in rural areas and the government's intention to consolidate the results of land reforms and boost agricultural production, rural areas and farmers had naturally become the focus of the healthcare policy. In June 1950, the National Rural Healthcare Symposium was held to solve problems in the rural healthcare system. Deputy Minister of Health Su Jingguan noted, "In the future, the focus of the healthcare sector should be on rural areas, while cities should focus on reforming old health facilities."[8] He asked healthcare practitioners to attach importance to rural health, eliminate the rural-urban gap in access to healthcare, and protect and promote the health of farmers. However, the country's general development plan released in 1953 for the transition period listed industrialization as the main task of the country, and the country's first five-year plan also focused on the development of heavy industries. The focus of the healthcare sector subsequently shifted. In January 1953, when formulating the annual work plan for cultural, educational and healthcare departments, the Cultural and Educational Committee of the Government Affairs Council pointed out that healthcare departments should

7 Report of the Party Committee of the Ministry of Health on the Task of Directing Healthcare Resources Toward the Countryside. In Department of Primary Care and Maternal and Child Health of the Ministry of Health, ed. *Collection of Rural Health Documents* (*1951–2000*) (p. 27).

8 Zhang Qin. On Rural Health – Report on Rural Health Symposium Held by the Ministry of Health. *The People's Daily*, July 25, 1950.

support industrialization and "focus on improving and establishing healthcare facilities in cities and mining areas and along transportation routes."[9] In October, the Party Group of the Ministry of Health reported to the CPC Central Committee that healthcare departments must increase support for implementing the country's general development plan. According to this report, given current situation in the country, healthcare departments should focus on improving access to sanitation in mining areas and access to healthcare in cities, combine rural healthcare initiatives with the rural cooperative and mutual aid campaign, and continue to advance the Patriotic Hygiene Campaign which aimed at preventing and treating the deadliest diseases in the country.[10] Since then, to align with the focus of the country's economic development plan, the healthcare sector had begun to concentrate on industrial areas while agricultural areas were neglected. Although the Ministry of Health later decided to attach equal importance to both urban and rural areas, the arduous task of industrialisation and the severe difficulties faced by the national economy at the time made it impossible. Lack of healthcare resources was still a major problem faced by the countryside.

2 Mao Zedong's Original Intention of Issuing the June 26 Directive

Mao Zedong devoted his life to liberating the Chinese people and improving their well-being. He attached particular importance to healthcare because good health is the foundation of happiness. As both his parents had died of illness, he was acutely aware of rural communities' lack of access to healthcare. The June 26 Directive was born out of Mao's concern for the health of citizens, condemnation of bureaucracy, and worries about the preparations against war.

As early as 1933, Mao Zedong pointed out when inspecting Changgang Township, "Disease is a big enemy in the Soviet area because it weakens our revolutionary power. It is the responsibility of every township Soviet to launch a public health campaign to reduce and eradicate diseases."[11] During the Revolution, which lasted more than 20 years, he attached importance to the construction of the Red Army Hospital, promoted the combination of TCM

9 Cultural and Educational Committee of the Government Affairs Council held a meeting to formulate this year's cultural and educational work plan. *The People's Daily*, February 3, 1953.

10 The Third National Healthcare Conference was held in Beijing and the guidelines and goals for the health sector were established at the conference. *The People's Daily*, December 31, 1953.

11 Mao Zedong. 1993. *Selected Works of Mao Zedong* (*Vol.1*). People's Publishing House. 310.

and Western medicine, and gave many instructions on healthcare and sanitation in the revolutionary bases. When the Chinese Communists were moving closer to the victory of the Revolution, Mao once again placed farmers at the heart of the cultural, educational, and healthcare initiatives. He said, "Eradication of illiteracy, universal education, popular art and literature, and public health are just empty talk if we leave out the 360 million rural population." When drawing up a blueprint for the country, he said, "We should actively prevent and cure diseases and promote universal health coverage."[12]

After the founding of the People's Republic of China, Mao Zedong participated in the formulation of the national healthcare policy, which pointed out the direction for the healthcare sector. In the name of the CPC Central Committee, he criticized public officials who neglected public health and demanded, "In the future, sanitation, epidemic prevention, and general healthcare must be regarded as a major political task, and we must attach great importance to this task."[13] The People's Republic of China quickly completed its first public health reform with his support. For example, Mao regarded schistosomiasis as a major public health problem in China. Schistosomiasis has a long history in the country. Before the liberation, 12 provinces, municipalities, and autonomous regions south of the Yangtze River, covering more than two million square kilometers, were affected by the disease. Patients with schistosomiasis reached more than 11 million.[14] Schistosomiasis destroyed many families and led to deaths. There were cases where it destroyed an entire village or township. The massive loss caused by the disease made Mao Zedong very anxious. In 1953, in a response letter to Shen Junru, Mao underlined the importance of stepping up the prevention and treatment of schistosomiasis. Under his instruction, in November 1955, the CPC Central Committee created a Leadership Group for Schistosomiasis Prevention and Control. Provincial, municipal, county, and village-level organizations were established in areas affected by the disease. A seven-year schistosomiasis eradication plan was formulated, including four years of intensive control and two years of winding up. The state put much money and effort in the schistosomiasis eradication campaign. On June 30, 1958, Mao Zedong spent a sleepless night writing a poem to celebrate the eradication of schistosomiasis in Yuyao County, Jiangxi Province. The publication of this poem not only propelled the campaign to reach a climax,

12 Mao Zedong. 1991. *Selected Works of Mao Zedong (Vol.3)*. People's Publishing House. 1078, 1083.

13 Mao Zedong. 1999. *Selected Works of Mao Zedong (Vol.6)*. People's Publishing House. 176.

14 Editorial Office of *Series on Contemporary China*, ed. *Healthcare in Contemporary China (Part 1)*. China Social Sciences Press. 2.

but also inspired Chinese people to make greater contributions to the development of the socialist country. In 1966, Mao instructed health facilities to offer free treatment for schistosomiasis.

It is precisely because Mao Zedong genuinely cared about the people that he criticized the bureaucratic working style of public officials. Pragmatism and strong awareness of service were crucial for health departments where a lot of intellectuals worked. Therefore, Mao Zedong was particularly concerned about the bureaucracy of health departments and the revolutionary spirit of medical staff. During the movements against the "three evils" and "five evils", Bai Xueguang, political director of the Department of Health of the Military Commission, pointed out the problems in the department's leadership. After reading the report, Mao Zedong said, "According to Bai Xueguang's report, the Department of Health of the Military Commission has not provided any leadership responsibilities concerning health related matters of the army. This is completely intolerable and must be rectified immediately." The report prompted Mao to question the effectiveness of the leadership of health departments. He instructed Xi Zhongxun and Hu Qiaomu to inspect the work of health departments at all levels of government. Mao noted, "Lack of leadership or political consciousness is unacceptable. Besides the Department of Health of the Military Commission, other departments might face the same problem. In this anti-bureaucracy movement, we must ruthlessly fight bureaucracy and build institutions that really work for the people."[15] Later, at the Third National Healthcare Conference, the Ministry of Health summarized the experience in the four years following the founding of the People's Republic of China, and reviewed mistakes relating to bureaucracy, subjectivism and decentralism.

In 1964, with the deepening of the Four Clean-ups Movement, Mao Zedong further underlined the importance of opposing and preventing bureaucracy and revisionism. In addition to criticizing cultural, academic, and educational departments, Mao was also angry that Beijing Hospital only provided services for senior officials. In June, during his talk with Vietnamese visitors, he criticized this phenomenon, berating Beijing Hospital for departing from reality, diverting from the mass line, and offering personal privileges to senior officials. On August 10, he wrote in his commentary on the *Report on Improving the Healthcare of Senior Officials* submitted by the Party Group of the Ministry of Health, "Beijing Hospital has many doctors and few patients. Bureaucracy

15 Mao Zedong. 1990. *Manuscripts by Mao Zedong after the Founding of the People's Republic (Volume 4)*. Central Party Literature Press. 176–177.

is wasting hospitals' resources. It should be open to the public."[16] Urged by Mao, the central government decided to abolish healthcare facilities set up for senior officials nationwide, cancel the system of full-time health promotion doctors and nurses, and ensure all hospitals were open to the public. In the June 26 Directive, Mao Zedong once again criticized the Ministry of Health for being bureaucratic, neglecting the needs of rural residents, and being disconnected with the grassroots and the masses.

The directive was born out of Mao Zedong's strong commitment to the mass line. It was not issued on a whim. However, let's revisit Mao Zedong's prior views about the international situation. We will find that the June 26 Directive is also closely related to his thoughts on preparations against war at the time. In the mid-1960s, China was in tense relations with many countries. Mao was alarmed over the increasing military threat from the United States and the Soviet Union. To the north, the Soviet Union continued to increase its military presence in the Sino-Soviet border region and in Mongolia. To the south, in August 1964, the United States began to bomb North Vietnam. In March 1965, the U.S. Navy deployed a large number of ships to South Asia, ready to attack at any time. American planes repeatedly intruded into the airspace over Yunnan, Guangxi and Hainan of China. In this context, Mao Zedong forecast that China was about to go to war and put forward the slogan "Prepare for war, prepare for famine, and serve the people". The Third Front Movement commenced. At the time, healthcare institutions were concentrated in the cities. Most medical staff were unfamiliar with the situation in the countryside, and the level of specialisation was very high in the healthcare sector. Mao was worried that they would not be able to cope with war. Sending medical professionals to the countryside to get in touch with the reality of Chinese rural society and help build rural healthcare facilities should be an important part of preparations against war.

3 Achievements Attributable to the June 26 Directive

After the June 26 Directive was issued, leaders of the central government, including Liu Shaoqi and Zhou Enlai, talked with employees of health departments to learn more about the situation, proposed specific requirements relating to the Directive, and urged the Ministry of Health to concentrate human, material, and financial resources in rural areas. One year later, the

16 Mao Zedong. 1990. *Manuscripts by Mao Zedong after the Founding of the People's Republic (Volume 11)*. Central Party Literature Press. 124.

June 26 Directive was publicly disclosed, which greatly encouraged most medical workers to devote themselves to the development of the countryside and boosted rural residents' confidence in the country's healthcare system. With the joint efforts of the central and local governments, urban and rural medical workers, and the masses, the rural healthcare system improved in leaps and bounds. Take the distribution of hospital beds, for example. In 1965, rural areas accounted for only 40 per cent of the country's total hospital beds. By 1975, this proportion had increased to 60 per cent.[17] Rural areas accounted for more than 65 per cent of the country's total health spending.[18] The June 26 Directive also effectively promoted the development of cooperative healthcare and the healthcare delivery model employing itinerant health workers, significantly improving access to healthcare in rural communities.

3.1 *Continued Development of the Healthcare Delivery Model Employing Itinerant Health Workers*

After the founding of the People's Republic of China, from anti-epidemic brigades who were sent to the affected areas to medical workers who visited the communities of ethnic minority groups to urban healthcare practitioners who went to the countryside to support agricultural production, the healthcare delivery model employing itinerant health workers had gradually taken shape. In January 1965, Mao Zedong instructed senior medical workers in urban areas to train doctors for rural communities. The Ministry of Health Party Group decided to make this a long-term mechanism. All medical workers with a title above attending physician, except for the elderly, frail and sick, were expected to participate in the itinerant health worker program at one time or another. Five months later, Mao Zedong issued "the June 26 Directive", promoting nationwide application of this model. Many medical workers went to live and work in the countryside and provided care for farmers in their homes or fields. Many well-known experts also participated in the program. In addition to providing medical services to rural residents, they also helped rural health workers to improve their skills. The trained "barefoot doctors" became the main actors in providing primary care to farmers. By the end of 1975, there were more than 1.5 million barefoot doctors and more than 3.9 million hygienists and birth attendants in production teams. More than 1.1 million medical workers in cities

17 National Bureau of Statistics. 2003. *China Statistical Yearbook (2003)*. China Statistics Press. 806.

18 Report of the Ministry of Health on the Barefoot Doctors' Work Meeting (Extract). In Department of Primary Care and Maternal and Child Health of the Ministry of Health, ed. *Collection of Rural Health Documents (1951–2000)*. 420.

and the People's Liberation Army participated in the itinerant health worker programs, and hundreds of thousands of urban medical workers decided to settle in rural areas. More than 70 per cent of graduates from medical colleges were sent to rural areas. More than 50,000 rural communes across the country, and almost every commune had set up a health center. This model remains in use. Other similar programs employed itinerant health workers, including Targeted Assistance Program, Bringing Culture, Technology, and Sanitation to the Countryside. The "10,000 Doctors Support Sanitation Work in Rural Areas" Project launched not long ago also adopt the itinerant medical worker model.[19]

3.2 *Rising of Rural Healthcare Cooperatives*

Rural healthcare cooperatives began to emerge in the mid-1950s. In November 1959, the Ministry of Health held a national healthcare conference in Jixian County, Shanxi Province, to introduce the practices and experience of healthcare cooperatives and asked all localities to adopt this model. After the June 26 Directive was issued, the Ministry of Health decided to run pilot projects in Macheng in Hubei Province, Jurong County in Jiangxi Province, Tong County in Beijing, and Xiangyin County in Hunan Province. The pilot projects provided a lot of meaningful experiences. At the end of 1968, Mao Zedong promoted the experience of the People's Commune of Leyuan County in Changyang County, Hubei Province in running a healthcare cooperative. He said, "Healthcare cooperatives are very good." Many newspapers, including *The People's Daily, Health News, and Red Flag*, published reports to promote this model. The national implementation rate has exceeded 90 per cent. Massive mobilization led to a dramatic rise in the number of rural healthcare cooperatives in 1969. By 1976, more than 90 per cent of rural communes had adopted this model. Healthcare cooperatives have met the basic medical needs of farmers at the lowest cost. Therefore, it is hailed by the World Health Organization as the only effective healthcare funding model for developing countries and has been promoted in developing countries as a model with Chinese characteristics.

After the reform, although healthcare cooperatives disintegrated after adopting the household responsibility system, the country still hoped to solve rural healthcare problems through healthcare cooperatives. In 2003, China began to pilot a new rural cooperative medical system. As of the end of September 2006, 1,433 counties, cities and districts across the country had adopted the new rural cooperative medical system, accounting for 50.1 per cent of the total number

19 Report of the Ministry of Health on the Barefoot Doctors' Work Meeting (Extract). In Department of Primary Care and Maternal and Child Health of the Ministry of Health, ed. *Collection of Rural Health Documents* (1951–2000). 420.

of counties, cities and districts in the country. About 406 million farmers participated in the new rural cooperative medical system, accounting for 45.8 per cent of the country's rural population, and the participation rate reached 80.5 per cent. From January to September 2006, 140 million farmers benefited from the new rural cooperative medical system and received a total of 9.58 billion yuan in compensation.[20] It should be said that the new cooperative medical care system is built on the practice and experience of healthcare cooperatives. Its background, popularization method, goals of supportive policies and the attitude of rural residents towards the system are directly related to healthcare cooperatives.

The June 26 Directive has left a mark in history with remarkable achievements and far-reaching influence. However, the "Cultural Revolution" broke out shortly afterwards. People made many mistakes due to the influence of formalism and dogmatism in implementing the Directive. Nevertheless, the merits of the June 26 Directive and Mao Zedong's commitment to serving the people wholeheartedly will never be obliterated from history.

20 Gao Qiang. *Comprehensively implement the spirit of the Sixth Plenary Session of the CPC Central Committee and develop a healthcare development model with Chinese characteristics – Speech at the 2007 National Healthcare Conference (January 8, 2007)*. Website of the Ministry of Health of the PRC. http://www.moh.gov.cn.

CHAPTER 16

Development of Home Care Services for Seniors in China

Li Wei and Ding Jianding *

Abstract

Since China promulgated its senior home care policy at the end of the 20th century, the perception of the term "senior home care" and the senior home care services in the country have undergone remarkable changes, with a significant increase in the methods of service delivery and related resources. China has developed senior home care standards to provide the norm for the sustainable development of the industry.

Keywords

senior home care services – social care for seniors – community-based care for seniors

Since[1] the adoption of the reform and opening-up policy, China has seen rapid economic and social development. This, coupled with the implementation of the family planning policy, made aging an increasingly prominent problem by the end of the 20th century. Senior care in China is gradually transitioning from the traditional family-based model to a new social support model. As the cornerstone of the senior care system, home care has always been the focus of China's efforts. It is also the answer to many problems in China's senior care industry. Home care for seniors refers to community-based in-home care services provided by the government or other entities or individuals to the elderly, including help with daily tasks, housekeeping services, rehabilitation care, and

* Li Wei, Ph.D. student, Department of Sociology, Huazhong University of Science & Technology, 430074; Ding Jianding, Professor, Department of Sociology, Huazhong University of Science & Technology, and Institute of Social Security, 430074.

1 This article is the output of one phase of the research project "Study of Home Care Insurance for Seniors in Rural China" (11BSH065) funded by the National Social Science Fund.

 | DOI:10.1163/9789004737990_017

comfort.[2] This article intends to explore the timeline of senior home care services in China.

1 Evolution of the Concept and Policies of Senior Home Care in China

1.1 *Evolution of the Concept*

Family care for the elderly has a long history in China. To look after the elderly in the family is deeply rooted in the cultural subconsciousness of Chinese people. Under the influence of a culture that respects the elderly, families used to be the sole providers of senior care, supporting the basic needs of the elderly such as food, clothing, housing, and transportation. Family support for the elderly is also enshrined in the Constitution of the People's Republic of China. For example, the third paragraph of Article 49 of the Constitution stipulates: "Adult children have the duty to support and assist their parents."[3] After China adopted the reform and opening up policy, with the socioeconomic transformation, Chinese families have also shrunken in size, and the percentage of nuclear families is increasing. In the meanwhile, the Chinese population is aging. Families alone can no longer effectively support the basic needs of the elderly.

According to the Principles for Older Persons adopted by the United Nations in 1991, older persons should "be able to reside at home for as long as possible" and "benefit from family and community-based care and protection following each society's system of cultural values."[4] Affected by changes in China's society and international policies, the senior care model in China is also changing. Under the new model, families continue to play a central role in senior care, but many other actors of society have also begun to contribute more to this process. On August 19, 2000, *Decision of the CPC Central Committee and the State Council on Strengthening the Work Related to Senior Citizens* set out the goal for China's senior care industry: The country should establish an senior

2 Office of the National Committee on Aging et al. Opinions on Comprehensively Promoting the Development of senior home care. Official website of the Ministry of Civil Affairs of the People's Republic of China. http://www.mca.gov.cn/article/zwgk/fvfg/shflhshsw/200802/20080200011957.shtml

3 The Constitution of the People's Republic of China. Official website of the Central People's Government of the People's Republic of China. http://www.gov.cn/gongbao/content/2004/content_62714.html.

4 United Nations Principles for Older Persons. United Nations For Aging. http://www.un.org/chinese/esa/ageing/principle.htm.

care system with community-based home care services at heart, supported by other actors of society, and the system should focus on providing social welfare, health care, sports, culture, education, legal services, and assistance with activities of daily living.[5] From relying solely on family support to combining family support and social support, the meaning of "home care services" in China has undergone a fundamental change in the early 21st century. It is widely agreed that engaging communities, NGOs, and individuals in providing senior care services is important.

1.2 *Evolution of the Policies*

1.2.1 Exploratory Attempts to Make Senior Home Care Policies

At the beginning of the 20th century, to better meet the aging population's needs, China began to roll out policies on a new senior care system that combines family support and social support. On February 13, 2000, to meet the Chinese population's rapidly growing demand for social welfare, the State Council forwarded *Opinions on Increasing Social Support for Social Welfare* issued by 11 departments and commissions, including the Ministry of Civil Affairs and the National Planning Commission, pointing out the overarching idea that "China should build a social welfare system with home care at the core, supported by communities and social welfare institutions."[6] This is the first time the Chinese government has used the term "home care (*jujia*)". It is China's earliest policy about senior home care. In 2000, Shanghai, Beijing, Dalian, Nanjing, Ningbo and other cities began to explore ways to develop senior home care.

Based on pilot projects across the country, the Ministry of Civil Affairs formally affirmed the status of senior home care. On March 5, 2005, it issued a *Notice on Launching Demonstration Projects for Specialized Senior Care*, proposing that China should build an elderly welfare system to support the basic needs of senior citizens. While the system is funded primarily by the government and collectives, private investment will become a new growth point. It will have home care at the core, community service as the basis, and specialised service providers as the backbone.[7] Since then, the status of home care services has been confirmed in various policy documents, including *Notice on Accelerating*

---

5 Decision of the CPC Central Committee and the State Council on Strengthening the Work Related to Senior Citizens. Website of the Civil Affairs Department of Hefei. http://www.hfgjj.com/n7216006/n7321984/n7327671/n7329259/9897347.html.

6 Opinions on Increasing Social Support for Social Welfare. Website of the Ministry of Civil Affairs of the People's Republic of China. http://shfl.mca.gov.cn/article/zcfg/200809/20080900019761.shtml.

7 "Notice on Launching senior care Social Support Demonstration Projects. 2005. *Social Welfare* 3.

the Development of the Senior Care Industry, *China's Eleventh Five-Year Plan for the Development of Senior Care*, and *Decision of the CPC Central Committee and the State Council on Comprehensively Strengthening the Coordination of Population and Family Planning Policies to Solve Population Problems*. Some provinces and cities have formulated relevant policies to support the development of the senior home care industry. For example, Shanghai has issued *Opinions on Further Promoting the Development of Senior Care in Shanghai*; Beijing has issued *Notice of Beijing Municipal Bureau of Quality and Technical Supervision on Launching the Senior Care Services Star Rating Campaign*; Liaoning Province has issued *Notice of Liaoning Provincial Department of Civil Affairs and Department of Finance on Further Promoting Senior Home Care*; Tianjin has issued *Notice on Promulgating 'Administrative Measures for Government Subsidies for Senior Home Care in Tianjin (Trial)'*; Shandong Province has issued *Opinions on Actively Increasing Social Support for Senior Care*; the People's Government of Nan'an District of Chongqing has issued *Opinions on Promoting Senior Home Care Services Across the District*. At the same time, 29 counties and cities/districts, including Hangzhou, Ningbo, Jiaxing, Jinhua, Taizhou, and Zhoushan, where conditions permit, are expanding the scope of their home care services programs to cover the rural elderly.[8]

1.2.2 Evolution of the Senior Home Care Policies in China

On January 29, 2008, 10 ministries and commissions, including the Office of China National Committee on Aging, jointly issued *Opinions on Comprehensively Promoting Senior Home Care*. This is the first policy rolled out by the Chinese government dedicated to this topic, marking a milestone in China's senior care policies. The document emphasizes the importance of senior home care, sets out crucial tasks and measures to support its development, and points out the industry's growth direction. It shows that China's senior home care regulatory framework was starting to take shape. Since 2008, the country has been working to institutionalize and standardize senior home care. Many provinces and cities have introduced policies to promote the development of senior home care comprehensively. At the same time, the central government has also strengthened its effort to provide guidance for the development of the senior home care industry across the country (see Table 16.1).

The Chinese government has also attached great importance to rolling out development plans for the senior care industry. On March 14, 2011, the Fourth Session of the Eleventh National People's Congress passed *the Outline of the*

8 Zhang Minjie. 2009. *A Study of Population Aging and the senior care System in China in the Past 60 Years*. Zhejiang Gongshang University Press. 221.

TABLE 16.1 Milestones in senior home care in China (2009–2010)

Date	Milestones
May 12, 2009	The Department of Social Development of the National Development and Reform Commission (NDRC) and the Department of Planning and Finance of the Ministry of Civil Affairs jointly held a conference in Nanjing to make arrangements for basic senior care pilot projects in 2009 and designated five provinces for pilot testing of the basic senior care system.
August 23, 2009	The Social Development Department of the NDRC, the Ministry of Civil Affairs, and the Office of China National Committee on Aging jointly held a conference in Mudanjiang, Heilongjiang Province, to discuss basic senior care pilot projects.
May 11, 2010	The Social Development Department of the NDRC and the Department of Planning and Finance of the Ministry of Civil Affairs jointly held a conference in Yichang, Hubei to decide for basic senior care pilot projects and officially designated 12 provinces, including Zhejiang, for pilot testing of the country's basic senior care system.
May 13, 2010	The Ministry of Civil Affairs and the NDRC jointly convened an expert panel meeting to discuss matters relating to the basic senior care system
November 7, 2010	The National Conference on the Progress in Building a Social Care System for the Elderly was held in Wuxi City, Jiangsu Province

SOURCE: FOR DETAILS, SEE THE WEBSITE OF THE NATIONAL DEVELOPMENT AND REFORM COMMISSION OF THE PEOPLE'S REPUBLIC OF CHINA, HTTP://WWW.SDPC.GOV.CN/GZDT/T20090519_279743.HTM; HTTP://WWW.SDPC.GOV.CN/GZDT/T20090831_298932.HTM, HTTP://WWW.SDPC.GOV.CN/GZDT/T20100514_346706.HTM THE OFFICIAL WEBSITE OF THE CENTRAL PEOPLE'S GOVERNMENT OF THE PEOPLE'S REPUBLIC OF CHINA, HTTP://WWW.GOV.CN/GZDT/2010-05/L3/CONTENT_L605751.HTM; HTTP://WWW.GOV.CN/GZDT/2010-LL/07/CONTENT_1740042.HTM.

Twelfth Five-Year Plan for the National Economic and Social Development of the People's Republic of China. On September 17, 2011 and December 16, 2011, the State Council released *Twelfth Five-Year Plan for the Development of the Senior Care Industry in China* and *Plan for Building a Social Service System for Seniors (2011–2015)*, stating that "senior home care services including help with daily tasks, housekeeping services, rehabilitation care, and comfort provided in the home settings of the elderly" and that "Relevant authorities should place home care at the center of the senior care system, focus on long-term care, rehabilitation care and community-based day care, improve the functions of different senior care institutions and facilities, and give priority to the most urgent needs of older people."[9]

Since 2011, following the release of the central government's senior care policy, local governments have begun to refine their senior care policies. For example, Sichuan Province has issued *The Twelfth Five-Year Plan for the Development of Senior Care in Sichuan Province*; Yunnan Province has promulgated *The Twelfth Five-Year Plan for the Development of Senior Care in Yunnan Province*; the People's Government of Xinjiang Uygur Autonomous Region has rolled out *Opinions on Accelerating the Building of a Social Service System for Seniors* and formulated relevant standards; Hangzhou has released *Standards for Community/Village-based Home Care Services for Seniors*; Guangzhou has promulgated *Measures of Provision of Community-based Home Care Services for Seniors*; Wenzhou has published *Senior Home Care Service Standards (Draft)*. Some local governments have also issued charging standards. For example, Beijing has released *Charging Standards for Home Care Services (for Seniors and the Disabled)*; Nanning City has issued *Home Care Service Charging Standards and Guiding Opinions*; the Municipal Civil Affairs Bureau of Shenzhen has released *The List of Designated Senior Care Institutions and Charging Standards for Senior Home Care in Shenzhen*.

In addition to assistance with activities of daily living, meeting the emotional needs of the elderly has also been enshrined in the country's law. On December 28, 2012, the amendment to the Law of the People's Republic of China on the Protection of the Rights and Interests of the Elderly was passed at the 30th meeting of the Standing Committee of the Eleventh National People's Congress, stipulating that family members should pay attention to the emotional needs of the elderly.[10]

Based on senior home care policies and senior care plans, we can see policy making relating to senior home care is led by the government and progressing gradually with the elderly in urban areas as its priority. China has rolled out basic policies for senior home care services. It is improving supportive mechanisms. Senior home care in China has entered a stage of standardized, all-around development.

---

9 Notice of the General Office of the State Council on Circulating *Plan for Building a Social Service System for Seniors (2011–2015)*. Website of the Central People's Government of the People's Republic of China. http://www.gov.cn/zwgk/2011-12/27/content_2030503.htm.

10 Law of the People's Republic of China on the Protection of the Rights and Interests of the Elderly. Website of the Central People's Government of the People's Republic of China. http://www.gov.cn/flfg/2012-12/28/content_2305570.htm.

2 Diversification of the Delivery of Senior Home Care Services and Increase in Resources

Since China began to implement the reform and opening up policy, with the introduction of home care, community-based care, and institutional care, the delivery of senior care services has been diversified, but family care for the elderly is still at the core of the senior care system.

2.1 *Continuous Diversification of Service Delivery*

2.1.1 Family-Based General Home Care Services

Although the decreasing family size has weakened the family's function in caring for the elderly, families still occupy a critical position in the senior care system in China. Assistance with activities of daily living and emotional support are two primary needs of the elderly. Spouses, children and other family members can effectively meet the needs of the elderly on these two fronts. The National Survey of the Elderly Population in China's Urban and Rural Areas (2006) shows that spouses were the main providers of assistance for seniors' daily living activities. Among them, the proportion of women who provided care for their spouses was higher than that of men. At the same time, most children could also provide assistance with activities of daily living, including assistance with shopping and accompanying seniors on medical visits. With respect to emotional support, family members or relatives can still effectively meet the emotional needs of the elderly. The vast majority of the elderly had access to spiritual comfort, such as companionship and heart-to-heart talk, provided by their family members or relatives (see Table 16.2).

As of the end of 2009, China had 18.99 million people aged 80 years and over, accounting for 11.4 per cent of China's elderly population (167 million). Most of them had moderate to severe disability. There were 10.36 million older adults with disability and 21.23 million older adults with mild or moderate disability in China.[11] Families alone could no longer meet the basic needs of the elderly, especially those with disability. The demand for social support for senior care was rising.

In 2006, the Chinese government announced the plan to build and improve a senior care system with home care at the core, and began to vigorously promote the development of senior home care.[12] *A Study of Home Care Services*

11 Pan Yue, Shi Yonghong, and Wei Minli. "To prioritize social care for seniors" is written into China's Twelfth Five-Year Plan as an answer to the question of how to care for 167 million older adults in China. *The People's Daily*, November 8, 2010, 13th edition.

12 Yao Yuan. 2008. Understanding the Chinese government's decision concerning senior home care from a macro-level perspective. *Population Research* 2.

TABLE 16.2 Provision of care and emotional support for seniors in urban and rural areas in China in 2006

Day care provider		Scope of services	Urban areas	Rural areas
Spouse	Female	Provision of care	65.7	71.3
	Male		40.1	38.7
Children Accompanying older adults on medical visits 89.7		Shopping	90.1	89.8
		90.6		
Emotional support			**Urban areas**	**Rural areas**
Ensuring older adults can meet or contact relatives at least once a month			87.9	88.8
Ensuring older adults have relatives with whom they can talk about their feelings at ease			86.2	87.1
Ensuring older adults have relatives who can offer a helping hand when they need it			83	86.3

SOURCE: ZHANG KAITI AND GUO PING. *THE BLUE BOOK OF POPULATION AGING AND THE ELDERLY IN CHINA* (*2010 EDITION*). 299–304
Unit: %

for Seniors in China's Urban Areas published by the Office of China National Committee on Aging in the same year shows that more than 85 percent of China's elderly population were willing to get home care services. About 48.5 per cent of the elderly population in China's urban areas had various care and support needs. Among them, 25.22 per cent needed housekeeping services, 18.04 per cent nursing services, 13.79 per cent companionship, and 2.25 per cent legal assistance.[13] Only 15.9 per cent of the respondents believed

13 A Study of senior home care for the Urban Elderly in China. Website of the Elderly Assistance Fund of China Ageing Development Foundation. http://www.capsc.com.cn/jijinhuipindao/laolingyinjui/2009-04-14/97649.html.

their care and support needs were satisfied.[14] Home care is undoubtedly an effective way to meet the care and support needs of China's huge elderly population, but its delivery should be more diverse.

2.1.2 Special Home Care Services Based on the Community

Communities are an extension of the family where elderly persons live.[15] Since home care services emerged in China, communities have provided crucial support. In 1993, 14 ministries and commissions, including the Ministry of Civil Affairs, jointly issued *Opinions on Accelerating the Development of the Community-based Care*,[16] setting out the goal of building a comprehensive, well-managed, high-quality community-based care network by the end of the 20th century with community organisations at the center, supported by various economic players. Home care is integral to community-based care, and communities are essential providers of in-home care services.

In 2000, Shanghai became the first city in China to launch a home care pilot project that relied on communities to provide daycare and door-to-door services for the elderly. In a sample survey conducted in 2006, 77.5 per cent of the respondents in urban areas said that their community provided at least one service for the elderly, and 57.4 per cent of the respondents in rural areas said that their villages provided care and support for the elderly.[17] Daycare is an essential type of home care service provided by communities. Community-based care makes up for the shortcomings in family-centric home care. Providers of community-based care can look after the elderly in the community during the day when family members of the elderly are not at home or do not have time. By 2010, China had built 12,000 comprehensive community-based care centres with daycare functions. In total, there were 12,000 beds for overnight care and 47,000 for day are.[18]

The Plan for Building a Social Care System for Seniors (2011–2015) released in 2011 pointed out that family services should focus on housekeeping, senior care,

14 Survey shows that only 15.9 per cent of the elderly population in China said their home care needs were met. Website of China News. http://www.chinanews.com/jk/kong/news/2008/02-21/1169860.shtml.

15 Zhang Kaiti and Guo Ping. 2010. *The Blue Book of Population Aging and the Elderly in China*. China Social Press, 304.

16 Opinions on Accelerating the Development of Community-based Care. Website of the Ministry of Civil Affairs of the People's Republic of China. http://zqs.mca.gov.cn/article/sqjs/zcwj/200912/20091200044461.shtml.

17 Zhang Kaiti and Guo Ping. 2010. *The Blue Book of Population Aging and the Elderly in China*. China Social Press, 306.

18 Notice of the General Office of the State Council on Circulating *Plan for Building a Social Service System for Seniors (2011–2015)*. Website of the Central People's Government of the People's Republic of China. http://www.gov.cn/zwgk/2011-12/27/content_2030503.htm.

community-based care and patient care, with targeted training provided for practitioners; it should continue to carry out rural community pilot projects and focus on the development of care and assistance for the rural elderly and other groups.[19] Community-based care has contributed to the development of home care services and diversified how home care services are delivered in China.

2.2 *A Remarkable Increase in Resources Related to Senior Home Care Services*

Families have always been the leading providers of senior home care resources in China. Alongside economic and social development, significant changes took place in senior care resources, and the responsibility for senior care no longer lies solely with families. Other members of society also shoulder certain responsibilities for senior care. Since the beginning of the reform and opening up, the rational allocation of government resources, neighborhood and community resources, and resources from the private sector have led to a significant increase in China's senior home care resources.

2.2.1 Family Resources

The shrinking average family size has led to a decrease in family resources for senior care. On the front of material support, with the expansion of social security coverage, the economic situation of older adults has greatly improved, leading to a drop in their economic dependence on the family. At the end of the 20th century, financial support from other family members and their own job pay were the main source of income for the elderly in China. According to a survey conducted by the National Bureau of Statistics in 1994, financial support for their children or family, their job pay, and retirement pensions were the three largest sources of income of the elderly. About 57.1 per cent of the respondents said financial support of children or family was their primary source of income. Only 15.6 per cent of the respondents said retirement pensions were their primary source of income. Most of the respondents who reported job pay as their primary income source were younger than others.[20] In the past ten years, the income of the elderly has increased significantly, and their economic dependence on the family has shown a downward trend. At the same time, retirement pensions have become the primary source of income for the urban elderly, while financial support from family members is still the primary source of income for their rural counterparts (see Table 16.3).

---

19 Notice of the General Office of the State Council on Circulating *Plan for Building a Social Service System for Seniors* (2011–2015). Website of the Central People's Government of the People's Republic of China. http://www.gov.cn/zwgk/2011-12/27/content_2030503.htm.

20 Du Peng and Wu Chao. 1998. Analysis of the Main Sources of Income of Older Adults in China. *Population Research,* (4).

TABLE 16.3 Income sources of older adults in 2000 and 2010 and urban-rural difference in 2010

Year	Region	Support of other family members	Retirement pensions	Job pay	Minimum living allowance	Property income	Other income sources
2000	Nationwide	43.8	19.6	33	1.6	0.2	1.8
2010	Nationwide	40.7	24.1	29.1	3.9	0.4	1.8
	City	22.4	66.3	6.6	2.3	0.7	1.6
	Rural areas	47.7	4.6	41.2	4.5	0.2	1.8

SOURCE: HAN YUMING AND WEI MINGYAN. ONLY MORE THAN 20 PERCENT OF THE ELDERLY MAINLY LIVE ON RETIREMENT PENSIONS. *THE BEIJING NEWS*, OCTOBER 23, 2010, A6-A7.
Unit: %

TABLE 16.4 Average family size in China (1953–2010)

	1953	1964	1982	1990	2000	2010
Average family size	4.33	4.43	4.41	3.96	3.44	3.10

SOURCE: CHAPTER 3 "POPULATION" (SECTION 5 "BASIC DEMOGRAPHIC DATA BASED ON SIX NATIONAL CENSUSES"). IN *CHINA STATISTICAL YEARBOOK 2011*. HTTP://WWW.STATS.GOV.CN/TJSJ/NDSJ/2011/INDEXCLI.HTM.
Unit: persons

As for assistance with activities of daily living and emotional support, the shrinking family size has led to a drop in the dependence of the elderly on the family. After the founding of the People's Republic of China, the average size of Chinese families gradually decreased, and a nuclear family, which consists of parents and their children, became the main family type (see Table 16.4). It has become increasingly common for older adults to live apart from their children. In 2010, 49.3 per cent of parents living apart from their adult children in China; of these elderly persons who are known as empty-nesters, 54.0 per cent live in rural areas, and 45.6 per cent in urban areas.[21] family structure and size changes have made it less likely for the elderly to obtain family resources

21 The 2010 Urban and Rural Elderly Population Survey Results Was Released. Website of the Ministry of Public Security of the People's Republic of China. http://www.mps.gov.cn/nl6/nl947768/nl950060/3331442.html.

for senior care services. However, in the short term, affected by the traditional culture, families are still the main provider of senior care in China, and family-centric home care is still the foundation of China's senior care system.

2.2.2 Government Resources

Government resources are crucial for the sustainable development of senior home care. Since the beginning of the reform and opening up, the central government has issued a series of documents and plans for developing senior home care, and local governments at all levels have also issued a series of supportive policies. These policies have pointed out the direction and facilitated the development of the senior home care industry. Under the government's guidance, China's senior home care services have grown rapidly.

1. Fiscal support. Fiscal support provides the funding needed for the sustainable development of senior home care. Governments at all levels provide support by purchasing services, setting up home care guidance or service agencies, and providing senior care subsidies. For example, since January 2008, the government of Shijiazhuang City, Hebei Province has been funding care services for "three-nos" elderly[22] and older adults who receive minimum living allowance; in 2002, the government of Pudong New District in Shanghai set up a non-profit district-level home care guidance center, and began to build home care centers and agencies in neighborhoods and towns within its jurisdiction; the government of Hailar District in Hulunbuir City, Inner Mongolia Autonomous Region, offers a home care subsidy of 60 yuan per month to all senior citizens over 60 years old who live in urban areas, have urban household registration, are physically unable or partially unable to take care of themselves and fall in any of the following categories: (i) people who are entitled to the minimum living allowance; (ii) people live in poor conditions and have no guardians; (iii) people who have been cited as model workers at provincial level or above; (iv) relatives of martyrs, (v) soldiers of with grade three or above disability; or (vi) older adults aged 100 years or above.[23]
2. Talent training. The goal of talent training is to provide human resources to support the sustainable development of the senior home care industry.

---

22 The "three-nos" elderly refer to older residents aged 60 years or above in urban areas who have no ability to work, no source of livelihood, and no guardian, or the guardians of whom are unable to provide care and support for them.

23 Summary of senior care Practices across China. Website of the Ministry of Civil Affairs of the People's Republic of China. http://fss.mca.gov.cn/article/lnrfl/zcfg/200903/20090310028387.shtml.

In the past ten years, in the face of the new situation and new targets concerning social management innovation and the social service system, relevant ministries and commissions of China have developed a blueprint for talent development in the senior care industry. In 2010, there were 113,000 social workers and 30,000 elderly caregivers in the social security sector, and the two figures are expected to increase to 1.5 million and 6 million, respectively, by 2020.[24] Support provided by the government on the human resources front is crucial for the sustainable development of the senior home care industry.

2.2.3 Neighborhood and Community Resources

The involvement of neighborhoods and communities has increased the accessibility of senior home care services. First, communities have built senior care facilities to ensure their residents can receive care at home. By 2004, China had built more than 30,000 Starlight Senior Care Homes to support home care and community-based care and provide venues for activities of older adults.[25] Secondly, communities have set up intermediary organizations and increased the resources of home care agencies. For example, Lvyuan District in Changchun City, Jilin Province have encouraged companies to provide paid senior care and housekeeping services for older adults; Xihu Neighborhood in Qilihe District, Lanzhou City, Gansu Province, has launched the Sunset Dining Table Program with the support of housekeeping service companies to provide older residents in the community with a full range of professional senior care services, including food delivery.[26] Third, communities have built information platforms and integrated home care resources. For example, Haigang District, Qinhuangdao City, Hebei Province built the Information Network for Residents in 2005 and set up information service centers in local communities, which provide 16 service items for older adults; in 2006, Kundulun District in Baotou City, Inner Mongolia Autonomous Region has joined hands with the private sector to invest more than 300,000 yuan in the first community service interactive platform

---

24 Notice of the Ministry of Civil Affairs on Circulating *Mid – and Long-term Talent Development Plan for the Country's Civil Affair System* (2010–2020). Website of the Ministry of Civil Affairs of the People's Republic of China. http://www.mca.gov.cn/article/zwgk/fvfg/zh/201110/20111000185430.shtml.

25 Speech by Minister Li Xueju at the Starlight Plan Review and Commendation Meeting & Tomorrow Plan Launch Event. Website of China's Social Welfare. http://shfl.mca.gov.cn/article/ldjh/200807/ 20080700017724.shtml.

26 Summary of senior care Practices across China. Website of the Ministry of Civil Affairs of the People's Republic of China. http://fss.mca.gov.cn/article/lnrfl/zcfg/200903/20090310028387.shtml.

in Baotou City, and established a district-level community rescue service system based on the telephone network and the Internet.[27] Finally, communities have supported the development of volunteers, which has increased human resources for the senior home care industry. Volunteers play an essential role in delivering senior home care at the community level and expanding the coverage of senior home care. According to data reported by urban areas in 2010, 2 per cent of the urban elderly had used in-home nursing services, and 6 per cent had used in-home medical services; data reported by rural areas showed that 3.2 per cent of the rural elderly had used in-home nursing services.[28]

2.2.4 Resources from the Private Sector

The involvement of the private sector has increased the professionalism of senior home care services. Because of the increase in senior citizens' demand for social care and lack of market access regulation, China's number of companies and NGOs engaged in providing senior care services has sharply increased. China now has many types of senior care organizations. As of the end of 2011, China had 2,503 public institutions providing care and support for the elderly, 19,407 centers providing legal assistance for seniors, 84,000 organizations engaged in promotion of older people's rights, 48,116 senior education institutes, and 413,000 activity rooms for older adults.[29] These organizations provide basic care for seniors. Companies, organizations and intermediary agencies have become major actors in China's senior care industry.

To meet the care needs of the elderly population, most local governments have purchased senior care services from private service providers. Companies, NGOs, and intermediary agencies participate in providing senior care services by signing contracts with the government. For example, the government of Daoli District in Harbin City, Heilongjiang Province have signed service procurement contracts with dozens of housekeeping service providers, real estate agencies, senior dating agencies and other well-reputed service providers for senior citizens.[30] NGOs also play an important role in the provision of senior

27 Summary of senior care Practices across China. Website of the Ministry of Civil Affairs of the People's Republic of China. http://fss.mca.gov.cn/article/lnrfl/zcfg/200903/20090310028387.shtml.

28 The report shows that nearly half of the elderly population in China live apart from their children. China Social Sciences Online. http://www.csstoday.net/Item.aspx?id=17071.

29 The Ministry of Civil Affairs releases the 2011 Social Service Development Report. Website of the Ministry of Civil Affairs of the People's Republic of China. http://www.gov.cn/gzdt/2012-06/21/content_2166922.htm.

30 Summary of senior care Practices across China. Website of the Ministry of Civil Affairs of the People's Republic of China. http://fss.mca.gov.cn/article/lnrfl/zcfg/200903/20090310028387.shtml.

care services. For example, the government of Haishu District in Ningbo City, Zhejiang Province has signed a senior care service provision and management contract with an NGO – the Starlight Association of the Elderly.[31] Intermediary agencies are also necessary providers of senior care services. For example, the government of Chang'an District in Shijiazhuang City, Hebei Province has collaborated with two highly reputable senior care agencies – Yiyangyuan and Shekang – to build community-based senior care centers.[32]

3 Timely Formulation of Senior Home Care Standards

Standardization efforts in senior home care began in the early 21st century. Now, China has released standards of social care services for seniors and professional standards for elderly caregivers.

The earliest standardization documents of China's senior care industry include *Standards for Building Design for Senior Citizens (1999)* and *Standards of Practice for Elderly Social Welfare Institutions (2001)*. Later, China issued more standardization documents related to senior care services, including *the Standardization Plan of China's Service Sector (2005–2008)*, *the Standardization Plan of China's Civil Affairs System (2006–2010)*, and *Notice Concerning the Standardization of Practice of Senior Care Institutions* issued by the General Office of the Ministry of Civil Affairs. Under the guidance of national policies, most provinces and cities have introduced local standards for senior care services and institutions. For example, Beijing has promulgated more than ten standards, including *Service Quality Standards for Senior Care Institutions* and *Star Rating of Service Quality of Senior Care Institutions*; Shanghai has formulated local standards for community and home care services for seniors; Jiaxing City in Zhejiang has issued *Fire Safety Standards for Social Welfare Institutions*.[33] These normative documents focus on the standardization of senior care services and the management of senior care institutions, especially in the three aspects of qualification, rating and demonstration. On July 20, 2011, the Ministry of Civil Affairs issued the Twelfth Five-Year Plan for the Standardization

31 Guo Qianghua and Yu Yaguai. 2010. Analysis of the Involvement of Non-governmental Organizations in Public Procurement of Services. *Journal of Southwest University for Nationalities (Humanities and Social Sciences Edition)*, (2).

32 Summary of senior care Practices across China. Website of the Ministry of Civil Affairs of the People's Republic of China. http://fss.mca.gov.cn/article/lnrfl/zcfg/200903/20090310028387.shtml.

33 Li Liguo's Speech at the 2009 Civil Affairs Standardization Conference. Website of the Ministry of Civil Affairs of the People's Republic of China, http://kjbz.mca.gov.cn/article/ldjh/201106/20110600159383.shtml.

of the National Civil Affairs System, proposing to formulate key documents for the standardization of senior care services during 2011–2015, which will greatly improve the quality and efficiency of senior care services and better meet the needs of senior citizens.

While strengthening the standardization of senior care institutions, China has also released professional standards for senior care service providers. In 2000, the Chinese government promulgated *National Professional Standards for Domestic Workers*; in 2007, the General Office of the Ministry of Human Resources and Social Security issued *National Professional Standards for Elderly Caregivers*, China's first standardization document for senior care service providers. On November 14, 2011, the General Office of the Ministry of Human Resources and Social Security issued *a Notice on Circulating Four National Standardization Documents Concerning the Profession of Elderly Caregivers* and revised *National Professional Standards for Elderly Caregivers*. Standardisation of senior care institutions and professional elderly caregivers has created a suitable environment for further industry regulation and laid a good foundation for senior home care service providers.

From relying solely on family support to combining family support and social support, the meaning of "senior home care" in China has undergone a fundamental change at the beginning of the 21st century. China's senior home care policies are affected by this change. After a period of exploration, China's senior care industry has entered the standardisation and all-around development stage. Its system is being continuously improved. China's senior home care resources have increased significantly, but families are still the primary providers of senior care services in China. Government support has improved the industry's sustainability, while the involvement of neighborhoods and communities has increased the accessibility of senior home care services. The participation of the private sector has increased the professionalism of senior home care services. Meanwhile, China has developed standards to provide a standardized framework for the industry's sustainable development.

Index

www.ingramcontent.com/pod-product-compliance
Lightning Source LLC
Chambersburg PA
CBHW071333230926
51849CB00002B/381
* 9 7 8 9 0 0 4 7 3 7 9 8 3 *

www.ingramcontent.com/pod-product-compliance
Lightning Source LLC
Chambersburg PA
CBHW071228230926
51849CB00001B/53
9789004707306